Making Sense of
Pensions and Retirement

Making Sense of Pensions and Retirement

John Lindsay
Head of Superannuation Department
British Medical Association

and

Norman Ellis
Under Secretary
British Medical Association

Foreword by
Mac Armstrong

Radcliffe Medical Press • Oxford and New York

© 1995 John Lindsay, Norman Ellis

Radcliffe Medical Press Ltd
18 Marcham Road, Abingdon, Oxon OX14 1AA, UK

Radcliffe Medical Press, Inc.
141 Fifth Avenue, New York, NY 10010, USA

British Library Cataloguing in Publication Data

A catalogue record for this book is available from the British Library.

ISBN 1 85775 090 X

Library of Congress Cataloging-in-Publication Data is available.

Phototypeset by Intype, London
Printed and bound by Biddles Ltd, Guildford and King's Lynn

Contents

Contributors

Mr Ray Henry
Superannuation Department
BMA

Mr Mike Rutherford
Managing Director
Royal College of Nursing Membership Services (see Appendix A for address)

Mr Peter Scott-Malden, CB
retired civil servant, a former deputy secretary
Department of Environment (since his retirement Mr Scott-Malden has developed a keen interest in the financial aspects of retirement)

Dr David Wells
retired general practitioner

Mr John Winn
Managing Director
BMA Services Ltd (see Appendix A for address)

Foreword

It is no exaggeration to say that for many of us the cash value of our pension at the time of retirement is often far greater than the value of our home. If only we spent as much care and attention looking after our pensions as we do on our houses! We ignore and neglect pensions at our peril. Far too often, we only attend to them when we are close to retirement and any options for improvement or change are largely closed.

This book has been written at a most opportune time. The NHS pension scheme is undergoing its most radical reform for many years. The effects of these changes are fully explained in the chapters that follow, alongside many other important topics relating to pensions and retirement. I advise strongly that this key book is kept close at hand, so that it can be referred to whenever pension problems occur.

Mac Armstrong
Secretary
British Medical Association
February 1995

Introduction

This book is relevant to anyone who is a member of the NHS pension scheme, whether a salaried employee or an independent contractor. The NHS scheme (which happens to be the largest occupational pension scheme in Europe) compares very favourably with other schemes. However, because most members are not familiar with its benefits, it is not usually perceived in such a positive light. It is precisely because of the scheme's considerable benefits, including the index linking of pensions, that it is important to treat with extreme suspicion anyone who tries to advise you to leave it.

Pensions – in spite of their importance – are widely neglected; most employees know little about their own occupational pension scheme and NHS staff are no exception. Pension matters are neglected because they can be difficult to understand, because retirement is regarded by many employees as a remote eventuality, and because the pension itself is often regarded as something which is immutable and not capable of being altered to any significant extent. Unfortunately, interest is often only aroused when retirement is imminent or when something goes seriously wrong, such as a bout of long-term sickness leading to ill-health retirement.

The book has been written to increase understanding and interest in pensions. We have tried to describe as clearly as possible the NHS pension scheme, using case studies to illustrate various pitfalls and problems. We have also described how it is possible for an individual to purchase extra benefits and have emphasized the need to start planning for retirement at an early stage.

This book is published at a time when pension schemes are subject to ever increasing strains caused by long-term demographic and social trends. Life expectancy continues to increase enabling retired employees to draw their pensions for an increasing number of years. The pressures generated by this demographic trend have been widely discussed in relation to the state pension scheme. These same pressures are being replicated on a smaller scale in many occupational schemes. Secondly, more people are retiring earlier than their normal retirement age. This is due to many factors including redundancy (both compulsory and voluntary), voluntary early retirement and the improved arrangements in many pension schemes for early retirement. Thirdly, virtually all occupational pension schemes are based on highly simplistic assumptions about what comprises the normal life expectations in respect of marriage, career and family. It would appear, not surprisingly, that almost all pension schemes are designed to cater for the male employee who works for the same employer throughout his career, is married with (preferably two) children, and whose death in retirement precedes his spouse. The pension rights of anyone who does not fit this actuarial straight jacket are adversely affected to an extent that broadly reflects the gap between their own life style and that of the actuarial model.

Pension schemes are gradually having to address the fact that only a small (and declining) proportion of their members actually fit this stereotype; most people change jobs at least once during their careers, most women have career breaks because of family and domestic commitments, and sadly a growing proportion of marriages end in divorce.

The NHS scheme is undergoing its most radical change for over 20 years. This March will see the introduction of important improvements to the scheme. Although they do not address all of the issues mentioned above, there has been some movement in the right direction; for example, the introduction of early retirement from age 50 (albeit with an actuarially reduced pension). The changes to the scheme are planned to take effect on 6 March 1995 in England and Wales, and on 1 April 1995 in Scotland and Northern Ireland. For reasons of simplicity we refer to 6 March in this book.

Finally, there are several people whom we would like to thank for their help and encouragement; Ray Henry of the BMA who checked the text for accuracy and clarity, Susana Salvo-Garcia also of the BMA, for help with various administrative tasks and Kathryn Shellswell for so patiently retyping a seemingly endless series of redrafts. We would also like to thank our contributors for providing their chapters.

As always we are responsible for the book's errors and omissions.

John Lindsay
Norman Ellis
British Medical Association
February 1995

Authors' note

This book does not and would not claim to provide independent financial and pension advice. Such advice must be obtained from accredited and reliable sources, which are registered under the Financial Services Act and are also knowledgeable about your pension scheme. Many professional organizations and trade unions provide an advisory service of this kind for their members. BMA members should not hesitate to contact BMA Services Ltd for financial advice and the BMA's Superannuation Department for advice on occupational pension matters.

1

An outline of the NHS pension scheme

Who can join? • Contributing to the scheme • The earnings cap • Scheme benefits • Protection against inflation: index-linked pensions • Maximum service allowable • Retirement • When is the best time of year to retire? • Payment of pensions and lump sums • Questions, problems and complaints

Who can join?

Membership of the NHS pension scheme is voluntary and is open to both NHS employees (including NHS Trust employees) and NHS practitioners, aged between 16 and 70 (Table 1.1). Prior to 6 April 1988, membership of the scheme was compulsory for eligible staff. The term 'practitioner' refers to independent contractors – GPs, dentists and ophthalmic practitioners – in contract with an FHSA or Health Board.

Table 1.1 Who is eligible to join the NHS pension scheme?

- Whole-time and part-time NHS employees
- General medical, dental or ophthalmic practitioners
- Assistant practitioners approved by the FHSA, engaged for three months or more, provided at least half the salary comes from the treatment of NHS patients
- Trainee practitioners
- Locum practitioners (but only if appointed by an FHSA or Health Board)
- Hospital locums
- Some scheme members who leave the NHS to work for approved organizations, eg hospices or university medical schools

Doctors and nurses employed by agencies cannot join the scheme.

Part-time staff

Part-time doctors have always been able to join the scheme. Other part-timers were not able to join until 1973. From 1973, they could join if working at least half time, and from April 1991 all part-timers have been able to join irrespective of the number of hours worked.

GP practice staff

GP practice staff cannot join the scheme at present. However, the government has agreed in principle that they should be permitted to join. The Health Department is surveying practice staffing arrangements to estimate the likely costs of the proposed change. The Department is also discussing with the BMA's General Medical Services Committee the financial and administrative arrangements for admitting such a large and diverse group of staff into the scheme. It seems unlikely that practice staff will join the scheme before 1996, if the government confirms that they can join.

Contributing to the scheme

Employees and practitioners contribute 6% of their salary (5% for manual workers), and this payment is subject to tax relief. The net cost to employees is further reduced because they are allowed a reduced rate of national insurance contribution. The overall effect of these two factors brings the real cost to an employee down from 6% to about 3% of salary. The employer contributes 4% of salary (5.5% in Scotland). In addition, the government meets the cost of increasing pensions each year in line with inflation.

How are these contribution rates set?

The contribution rates of occupational pension schemes need to be set at a level sufficient to pay for the benefits of the scheme. With most schemes, contributions are invested and the investment fund is used to pay benefits. The contribution rate is therefore adjusted up or down, depending upon the success of the investment fund.

However, the NHS pension scheme is only 'notionally' funded in this way. The contributions are not actually invested, but the Government Actuary's Department (GAD) makes a notional assessment of what the investment return would have been had contributions been invested. This assessment enables GAD to recommend a level of contributions sufficient to pay for scheme benefits. The employee then pays 6% of salary, and the employer pays the balance. The employer's share therefore fluctuates up or down, depending upon the success of the 'notional' investment fund.

The earnings cap

Since 1 June, 1989, new entrants to the NHS pension scheme (and all other occupational schemes) have been subject to an earnings cap. This means that they cannot contribute to or take benefits from the scheme in respect of income above a certain level. From April 1995, the earnings cap is £78 600. The government may increase it each year in line with inflation, but this is not guaranteed. Anyone joining the NHS for the first time after 1 June 1989 is subject to the earnings cap, as are any scheme members who preserved their pension benefits prior to that date and subsequently return to the NHS.

Anyone transferring between different pension schemes after 1 June 1989 will be caught by the cap, except for ex-NHS employees who transferred to the Universities Superannuation Scheme before 1 June 1989; they are not capped if they returned to the NHS scheme prior to 1 June 1994.

Members transferring from NHS to Trust employment will not be capped if their NHS employment commenced before 1 June 1989. Transfers between the NHS pension schemes in England and Wales, Scotland and Northern Ireland are not affected by the earnings cap.

Scheme benefits

The benefits available under the NHS pension scheme are described in later chapters (Table 1.2).

Table 1.2 NHS pension scheme benefits

- Pensions and lump sum (Chapters 2 and 3)
- Insurance and family benefits (Chapter 8)
- Early retirement (Chapters 9 and 10)
- Protection against inflation (Chapter 1)
- Buying extra benefits (Chapter 5)
- Mental health officer/special class status (Chapter 11)
- Injury benefit scheme (Chapter 8) (also available to non-members of the NHS pension scheme)

Protection against inflation: index-linked pensions

NHS pensions are increased in April each year in line with the movement in the retail prices index during a 12-month period ending the previous September. For those retiring during the 12 months preceding the April increase, the increase received will be in proportion to the number of months that have elapsed since retirement.

If an NHS pension is drawn before the age of 55, it is not increased until 55, at which point it is increased to cover the inflation that has occurred since the date when it was first drawn. However, ill-health, injury benefit and dependants' (spouses' and children's) pensions are increased annually, irrespective of the recipient's age.

Maximum service allowable

Scheme members can achieve a total of 40 years' reckonable service by the age of 60 and 45 years by the age of 65 (reckonable service is calendar year service, whether whole time or part time). Contributions can continue to be paid beyond the age of 65 up to the age of 70, providing that the maximum service limit of 45 years has not been reached. Special arrangements apply to members with mental health officer/special class status (see Chapter 11).

Retirement

Normal retirement age in the NHS pension scheme is 60; at this age, any scheme member may retire and claim benefits. However, it is possible to retire before the age of 60 under the following arrangements:

- voluntary early retirement (Chapter 10)
- ill-health retirement (Chapter 8)
- redundancy, organizational change, in the interests of the service or 'achieving a balance' (Chapter 9)
- mental health officer/special class status (Chapter 11).

Anyone still in service at age 70 must retire and take the pension and lump sum.

Scheme members are asked to give three months' notice of retirement; they should apply for retirement on a form available from employers and FHSAs/Health Boards and should take care to give at least the required amount of notice (see below).

When is the best time of year to retire?

Anyone contemplating retirement should consider the likely relative rates of salary increase and inflation over the following 12 months before choosing a retirement date. For example, if inflation is at a high level and the government has introduced a pay freeze, it would be advisable to retire sooner rather than later. This is because the pension in payment would be increased in line with inflation, whereas the salary paid in employment would not be increased and consequently would not generate a much larger pension. If the opposite circumstances prevail, ie high salary increases being awarded at a time of low inflation, it may be advisable to defer retirement.

Traditionally, salary increases and inflation normally move at about the same rate, and therefore the precise timing of the retirement date within a period of 12 months is not particularly significant. However, individual circumstances need to be taken into account, particularly since pension-able salary for employees is based on the best of the last three years of service. For instance, care should be taken when negotiating clinical direc-tor and medical director contracts and in assessing the effect of domiciliary visit fees (see Chapter 2).

If possible, NHS practitioners should retire at the beginning of a month rather than the end, because working for even one day attracts full dynamizing for that month (Chapter 3).

Payment of pensions and lump sums

The Paymaster General's Office (PGO) (see Appendix A) is responsible for paying pension benefits. The lump sum is entirely free of tax. Pensions are taxable and the PGO will deduct any income tax due.

The lump sum should be paid on the day following the retirement date.

Pensions are paid on the same day each month. The precise day will be chosen by the PGO to ensure an even spread of the huge number of monthly payments it makes (any arrears will of course be paid).

Box 1.1 Overpayments need to be repaid

Dr G's pension was a little better than expected. Unfortunately, it was also calculated wrongly, and the Paymaster General's Office took five years to notice. They had been paying Dr G £1200 per annum too much for this period.

To soften the blow just a little, it was possible to persuade the PGO to allow the doctor to repay the excess over the same period that it had been wrongly paid, ie five years.

From the BMA's files

It is important to give at least the required three months' notice of retirement to ensure that benefits are paid on time. If the required notice has been given, and the lump sum is nevertheless paid late, it may be possible to obtain an *ex gratia* payment by way of compensation. This would be based on the interest lost in not having being able to invest the lump sum for the period involved. It is more difficult to obtain compensation for late payment of pension, since it is assumed that because this would not have been invested if paid on time, no interest would have been lost. Any claim for compensation should be made to the relevant pensions agency (see Appendix A) in the first instance, although they may refer the matter to the employer or FHSA/Health Board (or to the PGO) if they feel that responsibility rests with them.

The NHS pension can be paid anywhere in the world and is increased in line with the UK retail prices index, irrespective of where the pensioner is living.

Questions, problems and complaints

If you have a question, problem or complaint about your NHS pension, assistance and advice may be obtained from various sources, including the following.

NHS employer or FHSA/Health Board

It is usually advisable to approach your employing authority or FHSA/Health Board in the first instance. They have the authoritative Employing Authority Guide produced by the NHS Pensions Agency to assist employers in administering pension arrangements. They also hold the documentation required to run the scheme, including application forms to receive or purchase benefits. They keep a supply of leaflets that describe clearly and simply various aspects of the scheme. They also tell members of any changes to the scheme.

The NHS Pensions Agency

The NHS Pensions Agency at Fleetwood, Lancashire (see Appendix A for its address) has overall responsibility for administering the NHS pension scheme in England and Wales. It retains a record of each member's superannuable service and calculates the benefits due on retirement. It provides helpful explanatory leaflets and answers questions about the scheme. Separate bodies administer the scheme in Northern Ireland and Scotland (see Appendix A).

Professional organizations and trade unions

If you feel that the information obtained from your employer/FHSA or the pensions agency is unsatisfactory or questionable, or an issue needs to be pursued on your behalf, your professional organization or trade union may be able to help. BMA members can ask its Superannuation Department for advice and assistance (see Appendix A for its address). BMA Guidance Notes on the NHS pension scheme are available from BMA local offices.

Occupational Pensions Advisory Service (OPAS)

OPAS is an independent and voluntary organization that provides free help and advice on occupational and personal pensions. This service is available to people who have tried unsuccessfully to resolve their problems with their pension scheme authorities. An OPAS adviser can be contacted through local Citizen's Advice Bureaux or by writing to the address shown in Appendix A.

Pensions Ombudsman

The Pensions Ombudsman is appointed under the Social Security Act 1990 to deal with complaints concerning occupational and personal pension schemes. The Ombudsman is completely independent and acts as an impartial adjudicator. The problem should first be raised with the pension scheme authorities concerned and, if satisfaction cannot be obtained, with

OPAS, before finally approaching the Ombudsman (see Appendix A for the address).

Compensation for administrative error

Although the regulations do not provide for the payment of compensation for administrative error, the pensions agencies will sometimes agree to make a payment on an *ex gratia* basis (particularly if there is a delay in paying the lump sum due on retirement, as explained above).

Box 1.2   *Ex gratia* compensation obtained

Due to an administrative oversight, an employer failed to deduct Dr P's added years contributions over a period of two years, by which time arrears of £5000 had built up.

The doctor was approaching retirement and it was not possible to pay these arrears back over a period within the limit of 9% of salary that attracts tax relief. However, the pensions agency offered to give the doctor full credit for the added years' purchase and to deduct the arrears of contributions from his lump sum on retirement.

This was a fair solution, except that it ignored the problem of tax relief. If the contributions had been deducted at the appropriate time, tax relief would have been granted. After a little persuasion, the pensions agency agreed that the amount of arrears payable would be reduced, by way of an *ex gratia* payment, to take account of the saving that the doctor would have accrued by way of tax relief.

From the BMA's files

NHS employees: their pension and lump sum

Calculating the pension • Calculating the lump sum
• Performance-related pay (PRP) • Medical directors of
NHS Trusts • Clinical directors

Calculating the pension

Like most other occupational pension schemes, the NHS pension scheme uses a conventional formula based on pensionable service and pensionable salary to calculate pension benefits; the following formula applies to all scheme members (apart from NHS practitioners; see Chapter 3):

$$\text{Pension} \ = \ \frac{\text{years of service}}{80} \ \times \ \text{pensionable salary}$$

Pensionable service

Reckonable (unscaled) service
The number of calendar years, months and days actually worked in the NHS count as reckonable or 'unscaled' service, irrespective of whether it is whole or part time.

Unscaled service is used for several important calculations, including:

- maximum service limits (40 unscaled years at age 60; 45 unscaled years at age 65 or beyond)

- the number of added years that can be purchased

- 20 years as a mental health officer, enabling doubling of subsequent service to commence

- the amount of additional service granted (ie enhancement) when retiring on the grounds of ill health, redundancy, etc (see Chapters 8 and 9).

Scaled service

However, it is 'scaled' service that is actually used to calculate the pension. Scaled service is unscaled service reduced to its whole-time equivalent (Table 2.1).

Table 2.1   Calculation of previous service for a person retiring on 31 December 1994

Period	Contract	Unscaled service		Scaled service	
		Years	Days	Years	Days
1.1.57 – 31.12.71	Whole time	15	–	15	–
1.1.72 – 31.12.79	$\frac{9}{11}$ths	8	–	6	200
1.1.80 – 31.12.86	$\frac{10}{11}$ths	7	–	6	133
1.1.87 – 31.12.94	$\frac{6}{11}$ths	8	–	4	133
Total		38	–	32	101

Thus, the 'scaled' service used for calculating pension will be 32 years, 101 days

Pensionable salary

This consists of the superannuable income paid to the employee during the best year of the last three years of service, based on the whole-time equivalent salary for the post.

Best year of last three years

These three years are calculated back from the actual date of retirement. For most people, the last 12 months of service usually produces the highest income of the final three years. However, this may not always be the case; for example, a doctor may have earned significantly higher income from domiciliary visit fees during one of the earlier two years.

Because of this method of calculation, it is not possible to receive the full benefit of any particular annual pay increase from 1 April (following the Doctors' and Dentists' Review Body recommendation) unless the employee continues working until the following 31 March, thereby completing a full 12 months at the new salary level.

Whole-time salary to be used

Whereas in calculating service (Table 2.1), it is necessary to scale down part-time working to its whole-time equivalent, part-time working makes absolutely no difference when calculating the salary component. The whole-time salary rate for the position is always used.

When is income superannuable?

Generally speaking, income is treated as superannuable if it is regular, likely to continue and relates to an employee's normal duties. Income is likely to be non-superannuable if it is irregular (eg bonuses), unlikely to continue and relates to work outside normal hours (eg overtime). Tables 2.2, 2.3 and 2.4 below show how income is treated for pension purposes.

Table 2.2 Superannuable income

Superannuable income includes:

- basic salary
- distinction awards
- London weighting allowance
- domiciliary visit fees
- associate specialist performance supplements
- additional NHDs up to whole time or maximum part time

Table 2.3 Non-superannuable income

Non-superannuable income includes:

- private income
- overtime or bonuses
- junior doctors' additional duty hours (ADHs)
- NHDs beyond whole time or maximum part time
- temporary additional NHDs
- income above the earnings cap (see Chapter 1)

Table 2.4 Income that may or may not be superannuable depending upon the employee's circumstances

- Performance-related pay
- Additional income from management posts, eg for medical directors or clinical directors

NHS practitioner income may be fully superannuable, partly superannuable or non-superannuable (see Chapter 3).

Calculating pensionable salary

The example in Table 2.5 shows how pensionable salary is calculated.

Table 2.5 Pensionable salary for a hospital consultant who has retired on 31 December 1994 (with no distinction award and no domiciliary visit fees in the final three years)

Period	Salary (£) per annum
1.1.94 – 31.3.94 $\frac{3}{12}$	49 680
1.4.94 – 31.12.94 $\frac{9}{12}$	51 165
$\frac{3}{12} \times 49\ 680$ =	12 420
$\frac{9}{12} \times 51\ 165$ =	38 374
Pensionable salary: 12 420 + 38 374 =	50 794

Bringing together pensionable service (see Table 2.1) and pensionable salary (Table 2.5), the pension is calculated as follows:

$$\frac{32 \text{ years, } 101 \text{ days}}{80} \times \ £50\ 794 \ = \ £20\ 493$$

Calculating the lump sum

The tax-free lump sum is usually three times the pension; in the example above, the lump sum would be: £20 493 × 3 = £61 479.

However, the lump sum will be less than three times the pension in the following circumstances:

* where a married man has reckonable service before 25 March 1972; this pre-1972 service accrues a lump sum at a rate of only 1 × pension. Service since that date accrues a lump sum at the normal rate of 3 × pension

- if a married woman nominates a husband who is financially dependent on her, because of permanent illness, for full widower's cover. In these circumstances, the lump sum is reduced for pre-1972 service in the same way as for a married man

- where a married woman opted (during the period 6 April 1988 – 30 June 1989) to provide a widower's pension for her spouse to include service before 6 April 1988; the lump sum is calculated by:

    pre-25 March 72   1 × pension
    25 March 72 – 5 April 88   2 × pension
    From 6 April 88   3 × pension

    Very few women took this option. From a life expectancy point of view, this makes sense because women tend to marry men older than themselves and to outlive their husbands. However, Chapter 18 gives additional comments on this important issue.

It is possible to avoid this reduction in the lump sum by paying extra contributions and purchasing an unreduced lump sum; this ensures that the final lump sum is 3 × pension. Chapter 5 explains how to purchase an unreduced lump sum and how much it costs.

Performance-related pay (PRP)

Whether any particular PRP scheme introduced by a Trust or other NHS employer is superannuable depends upon the nature of the scheme. The income from the scheme will need to be tested against the general principles explained above (see 'When is income superannuable?').

Because the PRP scheme for NHS managers provides for PRP increases to be paid within the scale maxima for the grade and for these to be consolidated into basic pay, they are superannuable. Any non-recurring PRP bonus payments paid over and above the scale maxima are not superannuable. On retirement, a further lump sum PRP bonus may be paid, which would otherwise have been paid for the last year of service. This is also non-superannuable.

If income from a PRP scheme is not superannuable, it can be made pensionable by paying additional voluntary contributions (AVCs) or free-standing additional voluntary contributions (FSAVCs). Chapter 5 provides details.

Medical directors of NHS Trusts

The superannuation status of income from a medical director appointment depends upon the type of contractual commitment. If the contract involves additional notional half-days (NHDs) beyond whole time or maximum part time, the medical director's income from this appointment is not superannuable. However, it is superannuable if:

- the additional NHDs do not take the doctor beyond the whole-time (11 NHDs) or maximum part-time (10 NHDs) limits
- it is paid as part of an overall contract that is also within the whole-time or maximum part-time limits.

When negotiating their contracts, medical directors should bear in mind that their medical director income, if superannuable, only generates extra pension if earned during the last three years of service. This is because their pension is based on the best year of the last three years' salary.

If medical director income is not superannuable, it is possible to use it to purchase AVCs or FSAVCs but not a personal pension.

Clinical directors

If a clinical director is employed under national terms and conditions of service, the appointment takes the form of 'temporary additional NHDs' (paragraph 14 of the national terms and conditions of service). Temporary additional NHDs cannot be superannuated because they are specifically excluded from the NHS pension scheme by the NHS superannuation regulations. The only exception is where temporary additional NHDs replace superannuable NHDs; in these circumstances, the NHDs remain superannuable and the clinical director's superannuable position therefore remains unchanged. However, the position is different again if the clinical director appointment is not made under the national terms and conditions of service. In these circumstances, the position is effectively the same as that of an NHS Trust medical director (see above).

The BMA's Central Consultants and Specialists Committee (CCSC) has produced guidance notes on medical director and clinical director appointments, which include advice on superannuation matters.

3

NHS practitioners: their pension and lump sum

Who can join the NHS scheme? • FHSAs and Health Boards • Calculating practitioners' pensions • Superannuable income • Dynamizing superannuable income • Calculating the pension • Calculating the lump sum • Non-practitioner service • Service before becoming a practitioner • Service after becoming a practitioner

Who can join the NHS scheme?

Although occupational pension schemes are normally only available to employees, the NHS pension scheme allows self-employed independent contractors to join. Their pension benefits are calculated in a quite different way from those of scheme members who are employees. For ease of reference, we refer to independent contractors as 'practitioners', as does the NHS pension scheme itself.

Practitioner membership of the scheme is open to:

- medical, dental and ophthalmic principal practitioners

- assistant medical practitioners approved by the FHSA or Health Board

- associate practitioners

- assistant dental practitioners (up to two per principal can join without the consent of the Dental Practice Board)

- locums appointed by the FHSA or Health Board (but not if paid by fixed weekly sum).

Trainee GPs and salaried GPs can also join the NHS scheme, but their employment is pensioned in the same way as non-practitioner employee service.

The following are not pensionable:

- locums not appointed by the FHSA or Health Board
- assistants not approved by the FHSA or Health Board
- doctors working under the retainer scheme.

However, the position of these doctors is under review, alongside the proposed inclusion of GP practice staff in the scheme (see Chapter 1).

FHSAs and Health Boards

For the purposes of the NHS pension scheme, the FHSA or Health Board (Central Services Agency in Northern Ireland – see Appendix A) assumes the role of the 'employer' in relation to practitioners; it maintains pension records and administers the scheme locally. If a medical practitioner is on the list of more than one FHSA or Health Board, one authority (the 'responsible' FHSA) assumes responsibility. Although these 'employer' administrative duties are actually undertaken by the Dental Practice Board for dentists (see Appendix A), for simplicity we refer to FHSAs and Health Boards when discussing the 'practitioner' arrangements.

Calculating practitioners' pensions

Non-practitioner (ie employee) pensions are based on a formula that takes account of the number of years of service and final salary. (This 'final salary' formula applies to most occupational pension schemes, whether public or private sector.) However, GPs' pensions are not based on a 'final salary' because their earnings tend to peak earlier in their careers, and in later years they may even drop as the volume of work decreases or because of a reduced commitment to the practice. A final salary scheme would be most disadvantageous if applied to these circumstances.

An alternative method of calculating pension benefits has been devised to take account of the fact that practitioner earnings may decline before retirement and is based on the total NHS superannuable income earned during a lifetime's career.

From time to time, practitioners have expressed concern that they may, as a group, be better off under a final salary arrangement. However, actuarial calculations (the latest being commissioned by the BMA in 1993) show that the method already used for practitioners remains the more favourable option.

Superannuable income

Since all superannuable income is taken into account when calculating practitioner pensions, the level of superannuable income is crucial. For pension purposes, practitioners' sources of income are divided into three types:

1 *fully superannuable payments*: these are regarded as consisting solely of net remuneration, and no deduction is made for expenses

2 *partly superannuable payments*: these are subject to a deduction to take account of the expenses element in the various fees and allowances. This amount is normally reviewed annually. However, in 1994/95, GPs received a phased increase as follows:

from:	Superannuable element (%)	Non-superannuable element (%)
1 March 1994	60.3	39.7
1 October 1994	61.5	38.5

3 *non-superannuable payments*: these are regarded as consisting entirely of the reimbursement of expenses.

Table 3.1 shows the superannuable status of various fees and allowances paid to medical practitioners (there are some variations for dental and ophthalmic practitioners). A limit is imposed on the amount of pay the Dental Practice Board may credit to a dental practitioner for pension purposes. This is revised annually and was increased to £75 000 with effect from 1 April 1994.

Dynamizing superannuable income

Because practitioner pensions are based on superannuable earnings received throughout their careers, it is essential that income credited each year retains its value, not just against price inflation but also against earnings inflation. The mechanism used to achieve this is known as 'dynamizing', which involves uprating the practitioners' income each year by a factor that reflects the annual Review Body award. These uprating factors are adjusted annually in line with Review Body awards. Their current levels are shown in Tables 3.2 and 3.3 (different figures apply to dental practitioners).

Table 3.1   Medical practitioners' superannuable income

Fully superannuable (100%)

- Seniority allowance
- Training grant
- Target payments
- Designated area allowance
- Inducement payments
- Transitional payments
- Course organizer training grant
- GP tutor income
- Hospital appointments (clinical assistantships, hospital practitioners, clinics, locums, staff funds)

Partly superannuable (60.3% from 1 March 1994; 61.5% from 1 October 1994)

- Basic practice allowance
- Assistant allowance
- Capitation fees
- Deprivation payments
- Maternity medical service fees
- Contraceptive service fees
- Temporary resident, immediately necessary treatment, emergency treatment, dental haemorrhage arrest and anaesthetic fees
- Night visit fees
- Capitation addition for out-of-hours cover
- Initial practice allowance
- Dispensing fees, on-cost, oxygen therapy service rents and fees paid for supply of drugs and appliances
- Postgraduate education allowance
- Students' allowance

continued

Table 3.1 *(continued)*

- Registration fees
- Health promotion payments
- Child health surveillance fees
- Minor surgery sessional fees
- Fees for vaccinations and immunizations carried out for reasons of public policy
- Rural practice payments

Non-superannuable

- Non-NHS fees:
    private patients
    insurance medicals
    sundry fees: cremations, private certificates, etc
- Payments and notional repayments under the schemes for rent and rates, and for ancillary staff
- Locum payments under the scheme for additional payments during sickness and confinement
- Prolonged study leave locum payments
- Locum payments for single-handed rural GPs attending courses
- Reimbursement for computing costs
- Associate allowance
- Doctors' retainer scheme allowance
- Net ingredient cost, container allowance and VAT paid in respect of the supply of drugs and appliances
- All payments (except the training grant) made in respect of a GP trainee
- Fundholding management allowance

Table 3.2 Dynamizing GPs' pay – uprating factors applied to superannuable pay

Year ending 31 March	Uprating factor	Year ending 31 March	Uprating factor
1949	25.129	1972	8.079
1950	25.129	1973	7.514
1951	23.246	1974	7.285
1952	23.246	1975	6.664
1953	23.246	1976	4.796
1954	23.246	1977	4.674
1955	23.246	1978	4.498
1956	23.246	1979	3.449
1957	23.131	1980	2.933
1958	20.997	1981	2.471
1959	20.707	1982	2.331
1960	19.797	1983	2.206
1961	18.929	1984	2.065
1962	18.929	1985	1.938
1963	18.929	1986	1.805
1964	16.603	1987	1.698
1965	16.603	1988	1.561
1966	15.095	1989	1.455
1967	14.029	1990	1.347
1968	11.322	1991	1.246
1969	11.097	1992	1.117
1970	10.473	1993	1.047
1971	8.727	1994	1.032
		1995	1.000

Table 3.3 Dynamizing dentists' pay – uprating factors applied to superannuable pay

Year ending 31 March	Uprating factor	Year ending 31 March	Uprating factor
1949	19.502	1972	8.047
1950	19.502	1973	7.414
1951	19.502	1974	7.065
1952	19.502	1975	6.468
1953	19.502	1976	4.899
1954	19.502	1977	4.802
1955	19.502	1978	4.674
1956	18.787	1979	3.562
1957	18.722	1980	3.027
1958	17.898	1981	2.551
1959	17.653	1982	2.407
1960	16.731	1983	2.278
1961	15.601	1984	2.133
1962	15.601	1985	2.002
1963	15.601	1986	1.864
1964	13.665	1987	1.754
1965	13.665	1988	1.613
1966	12.693	1989	1.503
1967	11.701	1990	1.391
1968	11.261	1991	1.290
1969	11.042	1992	1.159
1970	10.430	1993	1.045
1971	8.692	1994	1.030
		1995	1.000

Calculating the pension

Having dynamized each year of superannuable income, the dynamized years are added together to give a grand total of superannuable income earned throughout a practitioner's career. This grand total is then multiplied by 1.4%. The resulting figure is the annual pension payable.

$$\text{Total uprated income} \times 1.4\% = \text{pension}$$

For a practitioner retiring after 37 years in practice with a total dynamized superannuable income of £1 300 000:

$$£1\ 300\ 000 \times 1.4\% = £18\ 200$$

$$\text{Pension: } £18\ 200 \text{ per annum}$$

Calculating the lump sum

The normal method for calculating the lump sum is three times the pension (or 4.2% of the total dynamized superannuable income). In the example shown above, the lump sum would be as follows:

$$£18\ 200 \text{ (pension)} \times 3 = £54\ 600$$

or

$$£1\ 300\ 000 \times 4.2\% = £54\ 600$$

For married men with service before 1972, and for women who opted for a bigger widower's pension, the lump sum will be less than 3 times pension unless an unreduced lump sum has been purchased. Chapter 2 provides details of the lump sum accrual rates in these circumstances.

Non-practitioner service

GPs may acquire non-practitioner service in various ways, the most common being the mandatory hospital experience acquired before entering general practice. Many GPs also work as clinical assistants, hospital practitioners, GP tutors and course organizers.

Service before becoming a practitioner

If this service exceeds 10 years in calendar length, it will be pensioned as officer service (see Chapter 2). If it is less than 10 years, it will be pensioned as part of the practitioner pension, providing that this achieves a more favourable result than an 'officer'-type calculation; in most circumstances, it does. This service is incorporated into the practitioner pension by increasing the pension in proportion to the period of pre-practitioner work.

For instance, if the doctor shown in the above example worked for three years in hospital posts before becoming a GP, this would increase the practitioner's pension as follows:

Hospital service	=	3
Practitioner service	=	37
Total service	=	40

$$\text{Enhancement factor} \quad = \quad \frac{40}{37}$$

$$£18\,200 \text{ (GP pension)} \times \frac{40}{37} \quad = \quad £19\,676$$

$$\text{Pension} \quad = \quad £19\,676 \text{ per annum}$$

Service after becoming a practitioner

If the total 'scaled' length of this service is more than one whole-time year, it is pensioned separately as officer service (see Chapter 2). For example, a doctor working two sessions per week as a clinical assistant for six years:

$$\frac{2}{11} \times 6 = 1.09 \text{ years}$$

If the service is less than the equivalent of one whole-time year, the income is added to the practitioner's superannuable income in the year it is earned, dynamized and then counted towards the practitioner's pension in the usual way.

4

Practitioners: partnerships, retirement and other issues

Superannuable income: partnership shares • Notification of superannuable income • Tax relief on contributions • Forgoing tax relief • National Insurance contributions • GP assistants • The retainer scheme • Job sharing or part-time working • Retirement

---

Superannuable income: partnership shares

Unless a partnership requests otherwise, the FHSA or Health Board divides total superannuable income from general medical services equally between the partners. However, the partners can ask for their superannuable income to be divided according to their individual shares in partnership profits. Seniority payments can be treated separately.

Practitioners may also ask the FHSA or Health Board to take account of superannuable income received from other NHS employment (eg a clinical assistant post). Outside income of this kind is normally paid into the partnership and shared amongst the partners as part of the overall pool of income. However, contributions to the NHS pension scheme in respect of this source of income are paid solely by the partner earning it, who therefore receives any pension benefits accruing from it. If no further action is taken, the partner actually doing this work receives a higher overall pension (ie from both the GP and the hospital posts) than the other partners who are working solely as GPs. This potential problem can be overcome if the partners agree to adjust their partnership shares of GP superannuable income so that the other partners receive a higher GP pension, thereby equalizing pension benefits as between all partners.

Notification of superannuable income

Each year, practitioners are told by FHSAs or Health Boards how much superannuable income had been credited to them during the previous year, ending 31 March. (This information is provided on form SD86C.) The 'responsible' FHSA will do this for other FHSAs if the practitioner is on more than one list. Practitioners and their accountants should check this information carefully and raise any queries with the FHSA without delay.

Tax relief on contributions

GPs are in an unusual position in that, although they are self-employed, they are members of an occupational pension scheme. As a result, tax relief is granted on a concessionary basis (known as the 'A9 concession'). In addition to tax relief on the basic contribution rate (ie 6%), GPs are also entitled to full tax relief for any added years, unreduced lump sum or AVC/FSAVC contributions (see Chapter 5).

To ensure that tax relief is received on an actual year rather than a preceding year basis, the practice's annual accounts should show contributions separately in the current accounts of each partner, rather than as a deduction in the calculation of partnership profits. Tax relief on contributions should be claimed on the personal income tax return and not in the practice accounts or by a separate claim for personal practice expenses. It should be noted that the taxation arrangements of the self-employed will be radically changed with effect from the tax year 1996/97.

Forgoing tax relief

GPs are in a unique position in that they can renounce this tax relief, continue to accrue benefits from the NHS scheme, and then take out a personal pension plan (PPP) in respect of their NHS superannuable earnings, claiming tax relief on the PPP contributions instead. Details of this and other ways of improving pension benefits are discussed in Chapters 5 and 6.

National insurance contributions

Employee members of the NHS pension scheme pay reduced national insurance contributions because they are contracted out of the State Earnings Related Pension Scheme (SERPS). This also applies to any doctors working in general practice who are not self-employed, eg assistants or trainees. However, GP principals pay self-employed rates of national insurance contributions and do not benefit from the SERPS contracted-out national insurance reduction. SERPS and other State benefits are discussed in Chapter 17.

GP assistants

GP assistants may join the NHS pension scheme if:

• they are employed for at least three months

• more than half their salary comes from treating NHS patients

• FHSA or Health Board approval is obtained.

The FHSA or Health Board deducts the 6% employee's contribution from quarterly payments made to the principal, who should then recover this by deducting it at source from the assistant. The 4% employer contribution (5.5% in Scotland) is paid by the NHS rather than the employing GP principal.

The retainer scheme

Doctors working as GP assistants under the retainer scheme are not eligible to join the NHS pension scheme because their employment equates to less than the equivalent of three months' full-time employment in any 12-month period, which is the minimum employment requirement for assistants. However, their position is under review (see Chapter 3), along with that of locums and non-approved assistants.

Job sharing or part-time working

The level of pension earned by practitioners depends on the amount of superannuable income received throughout their careers (see Chapter 3). Therefore, the effect of job sharing or part-time working depends upon the extent to which this arrangement reduces superannuable income. Superannuable income will, in turn, normally be divided between the partners on the basis of their shares of the partnership profits (see above). It follows that the effect on the pension will depend upon the agreement reached between the partners on how profits should be shared among them, an agreement that will no doubt take account of any job sharing or part-time working arrangements.

Retirement

Normal retirement

Normal retirement age under the NHS pension scheme is 60; however, there is no obligation to retire at 60, and practitioners can continue to work and contribute to the scheme until the age of 70. Contributions to the scheme cannot be made after the maximum of 45 years' service has been completed.

Extension of pensionable age

Prior to 6 March 1995, if practitioners wished to stay in the scheme beyond the age of 65, they had to obtain prior approval from the FHSA or Health Board. This was known as an extension of pensionable age (EPA). The maximum extension was to age 70.

Practitioners had to apply for EPA before their 65th birthday, and FHSAs and Health Boards should have reminded them of this requirement three months before that date. The FHSA or Health Board had to obtain evidence that the practitioner's health was reasonably good and seek the views of the local medical committee. This information was then sent to the relevant pensions agency, along with the FHSA's or Health Board's own view of the application. If a practitioner retired after the age of 65, an EPA having been granted, any further practitioner service after this age was not superannuable. If EPA had not been sought, service after the age of 65 was not superannuable and the pension and lump sum was not payable until the doctor actually retired.

Box 4.1 Moving the goal posts

A GP continued working and contributing to the NHS pension scheme after the age of 65. His FHSA failed to remind him that he should apply for an extension of pensionable age beyond age 65, and the doctor himself was unaware of the need to do so.

Two years later, the FHSA realized its error and invited him to make application retrospectively, which he did. The pensions agency then refused the application on the grounds that the doctor's health was not good enough (an extension of pensionable age only being possible subject to evidence of good health).

The goal posts had been moved. The application was retrospective to the age of 65, when the doctor was in good health, yet his health was being assessed at age 67. After protest, the pensions agency relented and agreed that his pension scheme membership since age 65 was valid.

From the BMA's files

Temporary retirement

Practitioners have traditionally been able to retire for 24 hours and claim their pension and lump sum, having obtained the prior agreement of their partners and the FHSA or Health Board.

Changes to the pension scheme effective from 6 March 1995, however, abolish 24-hour retirement. The scheme now requires that there should be a genuine commitment to retire and that there should be a significant break in service, of at least one month, before returning to NHS work. The return to work may be on a full-time basis or on a reduced partnership commitment. The effect on the practitioner's pension of this return to work is discussed in Chapter 15.

Notice of retirement date

It is essential to give the FHSA or Health Board at least three months' notice of the intended retirement date so that benefits can be paid on time (see Chapter 1).

5

Financial planning for retirement: the NHS pension scheme

Is the NHS pension scheme worth 6% of salary? • How does this saving come about? • Opting out of the NHS pension scheme is a mistake for most people • Avoiding a refund early in a career • Can a refund be avoided? • Purchasing additional benefits • Contribution limits • Buying an unreduced lump sum • Purchasing added years of scheme membership • 'Old-style' added years • How many added years can be purchased? • What are the benefits of added years? • How much will these extra benefits cost? • Single payment • Paying by regular deductions from salary • Additional information relating to unreduced lump sum and added years purchases • AVCs and FSAVCs • Choosing which additional benefits to purchase

For most people working in the NHS, the NHS pension scheme provides the foundation for financial planning for retirement. It can ensure a good standard of living in retirement and compares favourably with other occupational pension schemes, in both the public and private sectors. In addition to its main components – the pension and lump sum – it provides other benefits, including insurance and family benefits.

Is the NHS pension scheme worth 6% of salary?

Most people are likely to feel that 6% of income (5% for manual workers) is a reasonable price to pay for financial security in retirement, particularly in an era when people are retiring earlier and living longer. Although the State pension must also be taken into account, it provides a relatively small income, which has been declining in real value and is not paid to men until the age of 65 (60 for women) (see Chapter 17 for details).

If 6% seems reasonable, 3% looks like a bargain; in fact, for most NHS employees, the real cost of the NHS pension scheme is closer to 3 than 6%, as the example in Table 5.1 shows.

Table 5.1   The real cost of the NHS pension scheme is closer to 3 than 6%

	Non-member		Scheme member		Saving
Salary		£23 325		£23 325	
Tax	(£4476)		(£4126)		(£350)
National insurance	(£2000)		(£1650)		(£350)
		£6 476		£5 776	
Net cost		£16 849		£17 549	£700
6% of £23 325	£1400				
less saving on tax and NI	£700				
Real cost	£700				
Real cost as % of salary	3%				

NB   Based on salary, tax and national insurance rates applicable from April 1994.

How does this saving come about?

There are two elements to the saving. First, pension scheme contributions are subject to tax relief and the individual's tax bill is reduced accordingly. Second, if contributions are paid into an occupational scheme, a reduced rate of national insurance contribution is payable (which is the case for most occupational schemes, including the NHS scheme).

Practitioners only save through the tax relief because they still pay the self-employed rate of national insurance contributions. Nevertheless, the tax relief saving alone reduces the real cost to well below 6%.

Opting out of the NHS pension scheme is a mistake for most people

Unfortunately, in recent years a very large number of people have been persuaded to opt out of their employers' occupational pension schemes and to take out personal pension plans (PPPs) instead. For the vast majority, this has been a serious financial error. In response to growing concern, the government asked the Securities and Investments Board to investigate the sales of PPPs, with a view to compensating people who have been wrongly advised. The Board's report was published in October 1994 and provides for people who have received poor advice to have their lost occupational pension scheme service restored.

For most NHS staff, the value and range of benefits available under the NHS pension scheme cannot be matched by PPPs, and they should not opt out of it.

The real cost of the NHS pension scheme to the member is much less than is generally believed. The employer (or FHSA or Health Board) contributes 4% of salary (5.5% in Scotland), which would not happen with a PPP. Because the NHS pension is index linked, it would retain its real value if inflation increased significantly. The government pays for this indexation. The government actuary has estimated that this costs an additional 6.4% of salary. These benefits would be lost if the member switched to a PPP.

The NHS pension scheme is able to restore lost pension rights to those members who have been poorly advised to opt out. However, this compensation will have to be paid for. Any person who feels that he or she has been poorly advised should consider approaching the company that sold the PPP and ask for compensation, and can also write to the appropriate regulatory authority. (If in doubt, ask the company for the name and address of the regulatory authority.) If necessary, one can write to the Securities and Investments Board (see Appendix A for addresses of the Board and other regulatory authorities). Finally, the trade union or professional association may be able to help in pursuing the claim for compensation. (BMA members should contact the BMA Superannuation Department.)

Although PPPs can contribute to retirement income, their role is usually limited. In most cases, it involves subscribing to a PPP in addition to (rather than instead of) the NHS pension scheme (see Chapter 6).

Avoiding a refund early in a career

A break in service can damage a pension, particularly if it occurs within two years of joining the NHS pension scheme. Scheme members with less than two years' membership who are thinking of taking a break (perhaps to travel or work abroad or to start a family) should take great care to preserve their accrued pension rights.

If scheme membership is less than two years, and the break in service is more than one year, members will normally be required to take a refund of the contributions paid into the scheme. Prior to 1988, a refund was payable if service was less than five years. In most cases, a refund is very poor value and should be avoided wherever possible. This is because:

- accrued pension benefits will be lost completely, and it will be necessary to start building these again on returning to the NHS

- the refund will be taxed

- national insurance contributions will need to be repaid out of the refund (this is because members of most occupational pension schemes pay a concessionary reduced rate of national insurance contribution).

These last two 'penalties' mean that the actual size of the refund received is disappointingly small, often far less than expected.

Scheme members with more than two years' scheme membership are not eligible for a refund of contributions; they must preserve their benefits by retaining them in the scheme, and these can be linked to any subsequent benefits that begin to accrue again on return to the NHS.

Can a refund be avoided?

Members may be able to avoid a refund even if their scheme membership is less than two years. A 'disqualifying break' can be avoided in one of the following ways.

- By returning to NHS superannuable employment within 12 months.

- By obtaining 'approval' from the NHS pensions agency for periods of work or study outside the NHS. Approved employment may be service in a developing nation or in some other employment that can provide valuable experience for future NHS work. Work in private hospitals will not be approved, but approval might be given for work in hospices or GP locum work. If 'approval' is granted, the period of 'approved absence' does not count towards the 12 months' qualifying break period. Thus, it would be possible to take a break of 20 months if at least eight months of this was 'approved'. 'Approval' should be applied for within three months of starting the period of work or study (see Appendix A for the address of the relevant pensions agencies).

- By taking unpaid leave and continuing to pay contributions.

- By continuing to pay contributions during maternity leave.

- By obtaining approval to discount a break caused by illness.

- By working in a superannuable locum post every 12 months. GP locum work is not superannuable (unless arranged through the FHSA or Health Board). However, 'approval' might be granted for such work. Hospital locum employment is normally superannuable, unless undertaken through a locum agency.

- By joining the Doctors' Retainer Scheme, if 12 months' service has already been accrued.

- By working for an organization governed by a 'direction' made by the Secretary of State under the relevant regulations. These 'direction' regulations cover medical schools in England and Wales, many hospices and certain other organizations. The effect of these is to enable doctors to remain members of the NHS pension scheme if they leave the NHS and become employed by one of these bodies. Details of organizations covered by a 'direction' are available from the pensions agency. Doctors working in universities in Scotland are only eligible if their contracts are for less than two years or if they are purchasing added years or the unreduced lump sum in the NHS scheme at the time of transfer.

Box 5.1   Avoiding a refund

Dr F had a break in service from 1973 to 1977, having had over four years' service up to that point. He faced the prospect of having to take a refund of contributions because his service was less than five years. He needed to obtain 'approval' of the 1973–1977 period in order to avoid a refund. Unfortunately, he had had substantial breaks from medicine during this period.

First, however, he was able to obtain approval for the period January 1974 to December 1975 when he was working abroad as a doctor. This still left the period January 1976 to June 1977, which was more than 12 months and therefore constituted a 'disqualifying break'. Happily, in the middle of this period, he had undertaken several weeks of valuable training which did qualify for 'approval'. The whole period 1973–1977 was therefore covered because no break was greater than 12 months, so Dr F was able to stave off the refund.

From the BMA's files

Purchasing additional benefits

Additional contributions may be paid to the NHS pension scheme to buy the following extra benefits:

- unreduced lump sum
- added years
- additional voluntary contributions (AVCs)
- free-standing additional voluntary contributions (FSAVCs).

Extra benefits can be particularly important to scheme members who were prevented from joining the NHS pension scheme until after the age of 20 (eg doctors who do not qualify until at least 23 years old) and therefore cannot otherwise achieve the maximum of 40 years' service by the age of 60.

In addition, income earned outside the NHS (eg from private practice) may be made pensionable by buying a PPP.

Contribution limits

Inland Revenue limits specify that tax relief can be claimed on only 15% of salary paid as contributions to an occupational pension scheme. Because the basic scheme contribution is 6% of salary, up to 9% of salary can be used to purchase additional benefits. However, PPP contribution limits are different (see Chapter 6).

Buying an unreduced lump sum

The tax-free lump sum available from the NHS pension scheme is normally three times the pension, but it is lower for married men with service before 1972 and for married women who have opted for a higher widower's pension entitlement (see Chapter 2).

It is possible to avoid this reduction in the lump sum by purchasing an unreduced lump sum, thereby ensuring that the lump sum is three times the pension. There are two ways of buying an unreduced lump sum: by a single payment or by regular deductions from pay.

Box 5.2   An interest-free loan

Dr H moved from the NHS to a university medical school but exercised his right to stay in the NHS pension scheme. Unfortunately, the medical school failed to note that he was paying extra contributions into an added years contract (see page 37), and for the next five years they failed to deduct these additional contributions.

Inevitably, this failure came to light, and a large payment of arrears was needed. Repaying these immediately would have involved a heavy financial burden and would also have breached the annual tax relief limit of 9% of salary. It was possible to agree with the medical school and the pensions agency that the repayment should be over a period of five years. This solution meant that the doctor was paying what he should have paid earlier, would receive his full added years credit at retirement and had effectively had a five-year interest free loan (admittedly offset by a considerable amount of stress in sorting the whole matter out).

From the BMA's files

Single payment method

The single payment method can be used within 12 months of joining (or rejoining) the scheme, and by newly married men (or women who have just nominated their husbands for a full widower's pension) within 12 months of their marriage. It only attracts tax relief in the financial year when the payment is made. This means that any payment that exceeds 9% of salary in that year will not attract tax relief.

The cost of this single payment purchase depends upon the number of years of service before 25 March 1972 (and the years of service before 6 April 1988 for women who opted for a higher widower's pension for this period) (Table 5.2).

Payment by deduction from salary

Buying an unreduced lump sum by regular deductions from pay involves entering into a contract that commences on a specific birthday and continues until the age of 60 or 65 (or 55 for those with mental health officer/special class status). Up to 9% of superannuable income can be used for this purpose, and this attracts full tax relief.

The cost of the purchase depends on the number of years that need to be purchased and the age at which the contract starts and finishes (Tables 5.3 and 5.4).

Table 5.2   Purchasing an unreduced lump sum by single payment

Service before 25 March 1972

Cost of purchase of one year of service prior to 25 March 1972 by single payment in respect of each £100 of current superannuable remuneration

Present age	Cost (£)	Present age	Cost (£)	Present age	Cost (£)	Present age	Cost (£)
25	2.67	30	2.46	35–44	2.35	49	2.46
26	2.61	31	2.44	45	2.36	50–54	2.47
27	2.56	32	2.41	46	2.38	55	2.48
28	2.51	33	2.39	47	2.41	56–57	2.50
29	2.48	34	2.36	48	2.44		

Service between 25 March 1972 and 6 April 1988

Cost of purchase to women of one year of service between 25 March 1972 and 6 April 1988 by single payment in respect of each £100 of current superannuable remuneration

Present age	Cost (£)	Present age	Cost (£)	Present age	Cost (£)	Present age	Cost (£)
25	1.335	30	1.230	35–44	1.175	49	1.230
26	1.305	31	1.220	45	1.180	50–54	1.235
27	1.280	32	1.205	46	1.190	55	1.240
28	1.255	33	1.195	47	1.205	56–70	1.250
29	1.240	34	1.180	48	1.220		

Purchasing added years of scheme membership

The added years scheme involves purchasing additional periods of membership and therefore benefits accrue in the same way as in the pension scheme itself, ie an additional index-linked pension and an additional lump sum that is three times the extra pension.

'Old-style' added years

The 'new-style' added years arrangements discussed below were introduced in 1983. Prior to that date, some scheme members purchased added years under the previous 'old-style' arrangements. For NHS employees, these accrue benefits in the same way as 'new-style' added years; however, for practitioners, 'old-style' added years can be identified on the dynamizing sheet in the year of purchase. In particular, many GPs

Table 5.3 Purchasing an unreduced lump sum by regular deductions from pay

Service before 25 March 1972

Additional percentage contributions required to purchase one year of unreduced lump sum for service before 25 March 1972

Age next birthday	Contribution at retirement age (%)			Age next birthday	Contribution at retirement age (%)		
	65	60	55		65	60	55
25	0.05	0.07	0.09	45	0.12	0.17	0.29
26	0.06	0.07	0.10	46	0.12	0.19	0.32
27	0.06	0.08	0.10	47	0.13	0.20	0.36
28	0.06	0.08	0.11	48	0.14	0.22	0.41
29	0.06	0.08	0.11	49	0.15	0.24	0.47
30	0.07	0.08	0.12	50	0.16	0.27	0.56
31	0.07	0.08	0.12	51	0.17	0.30	0.71
32	0.07	0.09	0.13	52	0.19	0.34	0.95
33	0.07	0.09	0.13	53	0.20	0.38	1.43
34	0.08	0.10	0.14	54	0.22	0.45	
35	0.08	0.10	0.14	55	0.24	0.54	
36	0.08	0.11	0.15	56	0.27	0.68	
37	0.08	0.11	0.16	57	0.30	0.91	
38	0.09	0.12	0.17	58	0.34	1.42	
39	0.09	0.12	0.18	59	0.40		
40	0.09	0.13	0.19	60	0.48		
41	0.10	0.13	0.20	61	0.61		
42	0.10	0.14	0.22	62	0.82		
43	0.11	0.15	0.24	63	1.23		
44	0.11	0.16	0.26				

bought 'old-style' added years at the first available opportunity in the early 1970s; the added years credited are shown on the dynamizing sheet for the year ending 31 March 1973.

Table 5.4 Purchasing an unreduced lump sum by regular deductions from pay

Service between 25 March 1972 and 6 April 1988

Additional percentage contributions required by women to purchase one year of unreduced lump sum for service between 25 March 1972 and 6 April 1988

Age next birthday	Contributions until chosen birthday (%)			Age next birthday	Contributions until chosen birthday (%)		
	65	60	55		65	60	55
25	0.03	0.04	0.05	45	0.06	0.09	0.15
26	0.03	0.04	0.05	46	0.06	0.10	0.16
27	0.03	0.04	0.05	47	0.07	0.10	0.18
28	0.03	0.04	0.06	48	0.07	0.11	0.22
29	0.03	0.04	0.06	49	0.08	0.12	0.24
30	0.04	0.04	0.06	50	0.08	0.14	0.28
31	0.04	0.04	0.06	51	0.09	0.15	0.36
32	0.04	0.05	0.07	52	0.10	0.17	0.48
33	0.04	0.05	0.07	53	0.10	0.19	0.72
34	0.04	0.05	0.07	54	0.11	0.23	
35	0.04	0.05	0.07	55	0.12	0.27	
36	0.04	0.06	0.08	56	0.14	0.34	
37	0.04	0.06	0.08	57	0.15	0.46	
38	0.05	0.06	0.09	58	0.17	0.71	
39	0.05	0.06	0.09	59	0.20		
40	0.05	0.07	0.10	60	0.24		
41	0.05	0.07	0.10	61	0.32		
42	0.05	0.07	0.11	62	0.41		
43	0.06	0.08	0.12	63	0.62		
44	0.06	0.08	0.13				

How many added years can be purchased?

The answer to this question depends on the amount of service that would have accrued at the age of 60, which is the normal retirement age of the scheme (different figures apply to those who have mental health officer/ special class status and can retire at 55) (Table 5.5).

Table 5.5 How many added years can be purchased?

Actual service (in years) projected to age 60	No. of whole added years that may be bought	Actual service (in years) projected to age 60	No. of whole added years that may be bought
39	1	23	17
38	2	22	18
37	3	21	19
36	4	20	20
35	5	19	17
34	6	18	15
33	7	17	13
32	8	16	11
31	9	15	9
30	10	14	7
29	11	13	5
28	12	12	4
27	13	11	3
26	14	10	2
25	15	9	1
24	16	Less than 9	Nil

What are the benefits of added years?

For non-practitioners, this depends upon service and salary, as explained in Chapter 2; for example, if during the period when the added years are purchased the scheme member is employed whole time then each added year would be worth $\frac{1}{80}$th of salary.

The example below shows the value of the purchase to a member who retires on a pensionable salary of £50 000 per annum having purchased five added years, whilst employed whole time.

$$\frac{5}{80} \times £50\,000 \; = £3125$$

Extra pension $= £3125$ per annum
Extra lump sum $= £9375$

For practitioners, the value of the purchase of 'new-style' added years will depend upon the level of dynamized superannuable income during the period of the added years contract. (Chapter 3 explains dynamized income and the method of calculating GPs' pensions.)

The following example shows the value of a purchase of five added years to a GP who earned a total of £450 000 in dynamized superannuable income during a contract that lasted 10 years:

Total dynamized income during period of purchase	£450 000
Annual average during period of purchase	£450 000 ÷ 10 = £45 000
Value of one added year	£45 000 × 1.4% = £630
Value of five added years	£630 × 5 = £3150
Extra pension	£3150 per annum
Extra lump sum	£9450

How much will these extra benefits cost?

The cost of purchasing added years is explained below. However, this cost is halved in respect of any members of the scheme who lost service as a result of taking a refund of contributions, if the lost service was:

• before 6 April 1978

   or

• as a GP principal.

Only this type of lost service can be purchased at half cost.

Single payment

This method of purchase can be used for up to 12 months after joining or rejoining the scheme. Tax relief is only available on up to 9% of salary in the financial year in which the purchase is made. The cost of the purchase by this method can be calculated by reference to Table 5.6.

Table 5.6   Contribution required to buy one added year by the single payment method

Age	Amount appropriate in respect of each £100 of annual remuneration	Age	Amount appropriate in respect of each £100 of annual remuneration
	£		£
20	25.20	45	20.10
21	24.70	46	20.30
22	24.20	47	20.50
23	23.70	48	20.70
24	23.20	49	20.90
25	22.70	50	21.00
26	22.20	51	21.00
27	21.80	52	21.00
28	21.40	53	21.00
29	21.10	54	21.00
30	20.90	55	21.10
31	20.70	56	21.30
32	20.50	57	21.60
33	20.30	58	21.90
34	20.10	59	21.90
35	20.00	60	21.70
36	20.00	61	21.50
37	20.00	62	21.30
38	20.00	63	21.10
39	20.00	64	21.00
40	20.00	65	20.80
41	20.00	66	20.20
42	20.00	67	19.70
43	20.00	68	19.10
44	20.00	69	18.50

Paying by regular deductions from salary

The cost of using this method depends upon the ages at which the contract to purchase added years starts and finishes. The completion date must be the age of 60 or 65 (or 55 for mental health officer/special class status groups).

Again, no more than 9% of salary can be used for this purpose, and these payments will attract full tax relief (Table 5.7).

Table 5.7 Contributions required to buy one added year by regular deductions from salary

Age next birthday	Contributions until chosen birthday (%)			Age next birthday	Contributions until chosen birthday (%)		
	65	60	55		65	60	55
20	0.36	0.50	0.61	42	0.87	1.22	1.83
21	0.38	0.52	0.64	43	0.91	1.30	2.00
22	0.40	0.54	0.67	44	0.95	1.39	2.20
23	0.42	0.56	0.70	45	1.00	1.48	2.42
24	0.44	0.58	0.74	46	1.06	1.58	2.69
25	0.46	0.60	0.78	47	1.13	1.70	3.02
26	0.48	0.62	0.82	48	1.21	1.85	3.45
27	0.50	0.64	0.86	49	1.29	2.03	4.02
28	0.52	0.66	0.90	50	1.38	2.25	4.80
29	0.54	0.68	0.94	51	1.48	2.53	6.04
30	0.56	0.70	0.98	52	1.60	2.86	8.05
31	0.58	0.72	1.02	53	1.74	3.26	12.18
32	0.60	0.75	1.07	54	1.90	3.80	
33	0.62	0.78	1.12	55	2.08	4.58	
34	0.64	0.81	1.17	56	2.30	5.77	
35	0.67	0.85	1.22	57	2.56	7.77	
36	0.69	0.89	1.28	58	2.92	12.06	
37	0.72	0.93	1.35	59	3.40		
38	0.74	0.98	1.43	60	4.10		
39	0.77	1.03	1.51	61	5.20		
40	0.80	1.09	1.60	62	6.97		
41	0.83	1.15	1.70	63	10.42		

Additional information relating to unreduced lump sum and added years purchases

These purchases can only be made if:

- the purchase contract starts at least two years before the chosen retirement age (unless the single payment method is used)
- there are no health reasons that would prevent the contract being completed (applications cannot be made during sick leave).

Payments by deduction from salary must continue until the chosen retirement age, unless this causes genuine financial hardship.

Insurance benefits

If a scheme member dies or retires on ill-health grounds before the age of 60, full credit will be given for the unreduced lump sum and added years being purchased, even though the purchase contract has not been completed (the only proviso being that the contract must have been in existence for at least one year at date of death or at the date an ill-health retirement application is made).

If the contract is set to run to the age of 65 and death or ill-health retirement occurs after 60, full credit is not given. The purchase is proportionately reduced and also actuarially reduced to take account of the fact that the contract has not been completed.

Part-time working

The credit of unreduced lump sum and added years that can be received will be affected by part-time working, because the level of contributions paid will be lower than that for full-time staff, and the income upon which benefits are based will also be lower.

What happens if the contract is not completed (other than for reasons of death or ill-health retirement?

Only that proportion of the contract that has been completed will be credited, and this will be actuarially reduced if benefits become payable early (eg on redundancy). If there is a break in service of less than 12 months, and benefits have not become payable, the contract can be resumed (although the amount purchased will obviously be less because of the missed contributions). The extent of any actuarial reduction depends, of course, on how long the unfinished contract has left to run before the birthday chosen for completion (ie age 55, 60 or 65) (Tables 5.8 and 5.9).

Table 5.8   Actuarial reduction: Added years

Whole years before chosen birthday	0	1	2	3	4	5	6	7	8	9	10	11	12	13	14	15
Percentage reduction %	0	5	10	15	19	23	27	31	35	38	41	44	46	48	50	52

Table 5.9   Actuarial reduction: Unreduced lump sum

Whole years before chosen birthday	0	1	2	3	4	5	6	7	8	9	10	11	12	13	14	15
Percentage reduction %	0	2	5	7	9	11	13	15	17	19	20	21	23	25	26	28

Applying to purchase the unreduced lump sum or added years

This should be arranged with the employer or FHSA or Health Board; a relatively simple application form has to be completed. It is advisable to apply at least two months before the birthday on which the contract is intended to commence.

AVCs and FSAVCs

Additional voluntary contributions (AVCs) and free-standing additional voluntary contributions (FSAVCs) are often termed 'money purchase' arrangements, because members' additional contributions are invested to build up a fund that is eventually used to buy additional pension benefits at retirement. The value of these additional benefits cannot be predicted and will depend upon:

- the success of the investment fund in the period up to retirement

- the annuity rates (based on interest rates) prevailing at the time of retirement: these determine the size of pension that the accumulated investment fund can buy

- the amount of charges and commissions deducted from the contributions.

AVCs

AVCs are an 'in-house' arrangement, organized through the NHS pension scheme. The Equitable Life Assurance Society (see Appendix A) has been chosen by the scheme to run the AVC arrangement. All occupational pension schemes are required to offer an AVC facility to members.

The scheme has negotiated competitive terms with Equitable Life for members to purchase these extra benefits. Administration charges are low and were further reduced from April 1994, and no commission charges are payable.

Details of Equitable Life's charges are shown in Table 5.10 (as a percentage of contributions paid). As far as investment performance is concerned, recent surveys confirm that Equitable Life is very competitive.

In views of these low charges and the good investment performance, the NHS scheme advises members that they are unlikely to obtain better

Table 5.10 Equitable Life: AVC administration charges

	When AVCs first introduced	From April 1994
Unit-linked contract	2.5%	1.7%
With-profits contract	2.0%	0.5%

value from FSAVCs (see below), the alternative type of money purchase arrangement.

FSAVCs

FSAVCs are not directly connected to the NHS pension scheme and are available from any company (banks, insurance offices, etc) trading in this field. Choosing an FSAVC provider is therefore a matter of personal choice for the member.

The following considerations might be taken into account in choosing an FSAVC provider:

- administration charges and commission payable; the provider should be able to explain these to you in simple and clear terms. They are usually heaviest in the early years, so early termination (or transfer to another company) of an FSAVC contract may be particularly costly

- past investment performance (although this can offer no guarantees for the future)

- the principal features of the contract (including any 'penalty clauses').

In view of the advice provided by the NHS scheme in respect of AVCs (see page 45), it may also be wise to ask your financial adviser or FSAVC salesperson whether you have been properly advised of the AVC and added years alternatives.

AVCs/FSAVCs: what benefits are payable?

As explained above, the amount of eventual benefit cannot be predicted. An AVC/FSAVC investment fund can be used to:

- buy extra pension for oneself

- buy extra pension for dependants

- buy a lump sum to be paid on death.

It cannot be used to buy a lump sum on retirement.

AVC/FSAVC pensions are not *automatically* index linked to the retail prices index. However, it is usually possible to take a smaller pension and for this to be increased each year by a specified amount (eg 3 or 5% per annum). Some companies, including Equitable Life, are able to offer full index linking, ie to cover any increase in the retail prices index. Again, the initial pension must be smaller to accommodate the extra costs incurred.

How are AVC contributions invested?

AVCs can be invested in one or more of the following three ways.

1   *With profits* (medium risk). This is similar to a with-profits insurance policy; bonuses are declared annually following the valuation of Equitable Life's assets and liabilities. These become guaranteed additions to the AVC contract. A final share of profits is allotted at the point at which the benefits become payable.

2   *Unit linked* (high risk). The contributions are invested in specific investment portfolios, and the value of the units purchased rises or falls according to the value of the underlying investment. There is a choice of investment portfolios, and the investor must accept the risk of market fluctuations inherent in this type of arrangement.

3   *Building society investment* (low risk). Equitable Life passes on the member's contributions to the Nationwide Building Society, which invests them in a special deposit account to ensure a secure return.

The choice of investment depends upon what priority a member gives to factors such as security, risk and likely investment returns. Although these choices are available from the AVC in-house scheme, FSAVC providers also offer a similar range of options.

Annual investment statements

Equitable Life advises members annually of the current value of their AVCs. FSAVC providers should have similar arrangements.

Why are AVCs/FSAVCs such a good investment?

Both AVCs and FSAVCs offer tax advantages that are not available with other forms of saving:

- contributions attract tax relief at the highest rate
- the investment fund is not subject to any income or capital gains tax.

However, the pensions resulting from AVCs/FSAVCs are, of course, liable to income tax in the usual way.

The open market option at retirement

At retirement, you are not obliged to draw your AVC pension from Equitable Life or your FSAVC pension from your chosen provider. Annuity rates are competitive, and it is often possible to obtain a higher pension from another company. This is known as the open market option, and it can make a substantial difference to the pension payable.

When are benefits payable?

AVC/FSAVC benefits must be taken at the same time as the NHS scheme pension.

How much can be invested?

AVCs/FSAVCs are subject to limits similar to those of the added years scheme; total contributions, including the basic NHS scheme contribution of 6%, must not exceed 15% of salary, thus leaving 9% of salary for the purchase of AVCs or FSAVCs.

However, there is a difference, in that for AVCs/FSAVCs the limit is 15% of taxable income, *not* superannuable income. This means that it is sometimes possible to invest in an AVC/FSAVC some NHS income that is not superannuable in the NHS pension scheme proper. For example, if a medical director of an NHS Trust works extra NHDs that are not superannuable under the NHS pension scheme, the income from this work can be used to purchase AVCs or FSAVCs.

AVCs/FSAVCs are subject to Inland Revenue limits on the benefits payable. Although Inland Revenue rules are complicated, the general principle is that total benefits (NHS pension, lump sum, added years and AVCs/FSAVCs) must not exceed the equivalent of a pension of two-thirds of final salary. If this limit is exceeded, the AVC/FSAVC surplus must be refunded and taxed at special rates (35% for basic-rate tax payers and 48% for higher-rate tax payers). Wherever possible, the AVC/FSAVC provider should ensure that these Inland Revenue limits are not exceeded.

AVCs/FSAVCs: employer contributions

It is possible for NHS Trust employers to make contributions to an AVC/FSAVC contract on behalf of an employee. This is not limited to a specific percentage of the employee's salary, but the limit of benefits not exceeding two-thirds of final salary still applies.

General practitioners' AVC/FSAVC limits

GPs can invest in an added years contract up to the equivalent of 40 years NHS pension scheme membership, but an AVC or FSAVC contract is restricted to the equivalent of 38 years and one month. This arises from technical factors inherent in the GP dynamizing method of pension accrual. GPs must be claiming tax relief on their NHS pension contributions as a precondition for entering an AVC/FSAVC contract.

Failure to complete an AVC/FSAVC contract

AVC/FSAVC contributions cannot be withdrawn. Benefits must be taken at the same time as benefits are drawn from the NHS pension scheme proper. The only exception applies to someone leaving the scheme with less than two years' service; as explained above, it is usually inadvisable to take a refund in these circumstances.

Anyone leaving the NHS scheme with more than two years' service will have the AVC/FSAVC fund preserved. This will remain invested and will be paid at retirement age (unless it has been transferred out of the scheme) (see Chapter 12).

If a member dies in service, the accumulated AVC/FSAVC fund is normally payable to the member's dependants.

Choosing which additional benefits to purchase

The available alternatives are:

- unreduced lump sum
- added years
- AVCs
- FSAVCs.

The unreduced lump sum purchase is only available to (and necessary for) certain groups, particularly married men with service before 1972. In most cases, it is a good investment because the investment itself attracts tax relief and the benefit created (the extra lump sum) is entirely free of tax.

The choice between added years, AVCs and FSAVCs depends upon a variety of factors including:

- age
- attitudes towards investment risk
- attitudes towards likely future inflation rates
- future career plans
- insurance needs (ill health, death in service)
- flexibility requirements
- charges and commissions payable.

The choice of investment must, of course, be the individual's own decision, and the information provided above may be sufficient to enable this choice to be made. However, members may wish to seek independent financial advice if they need further information before taking an important decision that is difficult to reverse. It must be kept in mind that substantial commissions are payable to anyone selling an FSAVC but that they will receive nothing if they recommend added years or AVCs, unless the prospective purchaser is paying an agreed fee for advice. Be sure that the adviser presents all the options, in a balanced way. Doctors who are BMA members may seek independent financial advice from BMA Services Ltd (see Appendix A).

Table 5.11 below summarizes some aspects that might be taken into account. It should not be regarded as an alternative to considering carefully the key factors that are likely to influence any individual's choice.

Table 5.11 Summary of features: added years/AVCs/FSAVCs

Scheme feature	Added years	AVCs	FSAVC
Contributions	Cannot vary	Variable and flexible	Variable and flexible
Benefit limits	40 years at age 60	Equivalent of 40 years at age 60 (38.1 years for GP)	Equivalent of 40 years at age 60 (38.1 years for GP)
GPs not claiming tax relief	Available	Not available	Not available
Widows'/ widowers'* and children's benefits	Available at no extra cost*	Available at extra cost	Available at extra cost
Death in service/ill-health benefits	Service may be enhanced	Based on size of fund	Based on size of fund
Extra lump sum	Three times extra pension	Not available	Not available
Indexing of pension	Linked to retail prices index	Available with lower pension	Possibly available with lower pension
Tax relief on contributions	Must not exceed 15% of superannuable income	Must not exceed 15% of taxable income	Must not exceed 15% of taxable income
Dependent upon investment returns	No	Yes	Yes
Dependent upon annuity rates at retirement	No	Yes	Yes
Charges and commissions payable	None	Low	Take care

* Widowers from 6 April 1988.

6

Financial planning for retirement: personal pensions

What income can be pensioned through a PPP?
• Contributions • Benefits • Insurance • Choices on retirement • Choosing a PPP scheme • What type of investment is best? • General practitioners

Personal pension plans (PPPs) were introduced in 1988. They are quite distinct from occupational pension schemes, including the NHS scheme, and may be of value to anyone who cannot join an occupational scheme or has private earned income over and above their NHS income that is not pensionable within the NHS scheme.

PPPs are similar to occupational pension schemes in the sense that they both attract tax relief on contributions and are both designed to yield a pension, and lump sum, at retirement. PPPs are an attractive investment, because of both the tax relief on contributions and the fact that the investment fund grows entirely free of capital gains tax.

As explained in Chapter 5, it is not financially wise for most people to opt out of their occupational pension scheme simply in order to start a PPP. PPPs must be regarded as no more than a supplement to the NHS pension scheme.

What income can be pensioned through a PPP?

Salaried NHS staff who are in the NHS pension scheme can take out a PPP to cover any private income. It is also theoretically possible to opt out of the NHS scheme in respect of employment with one NHS employer, whilst staying in the scheme in respect of separate concurrent employment with another NHS employer. Under this arrangement, a PPP can apply to the opted-out post. However, as explained above, any decision to opt out must be given very careful consideration.

Other NHS income coming from the same employer cannot be made pensionable in a PPP even if it is not superannuable within the NHS pension scheme (typical examples of which include junior doctors' additional duty hours (ADHs), extra notional half-days (NHDs) above whole time or maximum part time, etc). However, it may be possible to make these sources of income pensionable by means of additional voluntary contributions (AVCs) or free-standing additional voluntary contributions (FSAVCs) (see Chapter 5).

The earnings cap limit, which is currently £78 600 (see Chapter 1), is applied separately to PPPs and occupational pension schemes; private earnings up to a limit of £78 600 can be pensioned separately through a PPP.

Contributions

Unlike occupational pension schemes, where the Inland Revenue imposes a strict limit on how much benefit can be paid out (in short the pension and lump sum taken together must exceed no more than two-thirds of final salary), there is no limit on how much benefit can be derived from a PPP. However, there are limits on how much money can be invested in a PPP.

The amount of contribution (as a percentage of income) that can be paid into a PPP depends upon age (Table 6.1). Tax relief is available up to these limits; for example, at age 47 it is possible to obtain tax relief on 25% of annual income invested in a PPP.

Table 6.1   Percentage of income that can be invested in a PPP

Age	% of income
35 or less	17.5
36–45	20.0
46–50	25.0
51–55	30.0
56–60	35.0
61 and over	40.0

Benefits

PPPs are a 'money purchase' arrangement, ie their benefits do not depend on some specific proportion of salary, as is the case with most occupational schemes (eg $\frac{1}{80}$th of salary per year of service). Instead, ultimate benefits simply reflect the amount of money invested and the success of the investment fund. Thus, the amount of benefit eventually earned depends upon several factors, including:

- the amount of money paid into the PPP. This depends upon the investor's income level and whether he or she is prepared to invest the maximum allowable percentage of income (Table 6.1)

- the age at which the PPP starts. This determines both the percentage of income that can be invested and the length of time it is invested (ie the younger the entry age, the more time the investment has to grow)

- the age at which the pension is drawn. Although a personal pension may be drawn from the age of 50 onwards, the earlier it is drawn, the lower its value. This is because it has had less time to accrue and has to be payable for a longer life span

- the level of annuity rates (ie interest rates) prevailing when the pension starts. If interest rates are high, the accumulated PPP investment fund can buy a relatively higher annuity (ie pension). The reverse also applies: low interest rates mean lower annuities. This can significantly affect the pension received and should be taken into account when choosing a retirement date. Legislation is in the pipeline which will enable the lump sum to be taken but to defer the purchase of an annuity, with a view to taking advantage of any future rise in interest rates

- the success of the investment; there are a number of different types of investment and investment management arrangements from which to choose. The higher the investment returns on the fund, the higher the eventual pension paid

- the amount of charges and commissions payable.

The pension can be taken at any time between the ages of 50 and 75. It is not necessary to retire from a post, or to take the personal pension when taking the NHS pension.

Once a date is chosen, 25% of the accumulated PPP investment fund may be taken as a tax-free lump sum. The balance of the fund must be used to purchase a pension (an annuity). This is known as a 'compulsory purchase' annuity, and income from it is subject to income tax in the normal way. However, if the tax-free lump sum is used to purchase an additional annuity, this is treated differently for tax purposes. This is known as a 'purchased life' annuity and it is only partially taxed, because the tax authorities regard it as comprising two elements: one part is normal taxable income, whereas the remainder is deemed to be a return of the tax-free lump sum and is therefore not taxable.

Insurance

It is possible to take out life assurance as part of the PPP; tax relief is allowed for this purpose on up to 5% of income (within the overall PPP contribution limits). It is also possible to arrange for any lump sum death benefit to be put in trust for a member's children or other dependants, thereby ensuring that it is not part of the estate for inheritance tax purposes.

It may be possible to draw a PPP early on the grounds of ill health; however, it is important to check whether or not any penalties will be imposed. The need for ill-health cover depends on the level of ill-health retirement benefits a member can expect from the NHS scheme on ill-health retirement (see Chapter 8), or from any other insurance cover.

Choices on retirement

There is no obligation to draw a PPP-based pension from the PPP provider, ie the company that has invested the contributions. They may not be able to provide the most competitive annuity rate. In these circumstances, the 'open market option' may be used to find out what annuity rates are offered by other companies and to choose the one that offers the best value. This is a very valuable option, because annuity rates are competitive and can significantly affect pensions.

Most people draw the maximum available tax-free lump sum (ie 25% of the investment fund). This lump sum can, if desired, be used to purchase an annuity (pension) as explained when discussing 'purchased life' annuities above. The balance of the PPP fund (ie 75%) must be used to purchase a pension or annuity. When purchasing this pension, the following options are available:

- it can be set at the highest possible level of pension without any provision for future increases or survivors' benefits

- it can provide a pension that is increased annually, for example at 3 or 5% per year

- there may be a joint life pension, a proportion being paid to the spouse on the death of the scheme member

- it may be a guaranteed term pension, so that a minimum number of years of benefit (eg 5) is paid even if the scheme member dies.

The actual amount of pension depends on which option is chosen: extra benefits (eg annual increases or survivors' pensions) must be paid for by a lower level of pension being drawn at the outset.

Choosing a PPP scheme

PPPs may be bought from many sources, including banks, building societies and insurance companies.

Although it is not possible to predict future returns on investments, it is usually advisable to choose a reputable company that has had a record of good investment returns.

Another important factor is the charges levied on purchase of a PPP. Charging structures are difficult to understand, varying widely and being applied in different ways, and charges can eat up a sizeable portion of the contributions. They tend to be higher in the early years of the PPP and can have a significant impact if the PPP is cancelled or transferred soon after commencement.

It is usually advisable to obtain assistance from a reputable independent financial adviser, who should be able to review a variety of schemes and explain charging structures. BMA members can obtain independent financial advice from BMA Services Ltd (see Appendix A).

What type of investment is best?

PPP schemes offer a variety of investment options.

Deposit-based investments

These are similar to ordinary savings accounts; the capital sum cannot fall and interest is added to it at the prevailing rates.

With-profits investments

With-profits investments guarantee a specific level of pension on retirement. Bonuses are added regularly to the accruing capital sum; once paid, these cannot be withdrawn. An end-point (ie terminal) bonus is usually added when the pension is drawn. The level of these bonuses depends upon both the success of the capital investment fund and other factors, such as the company's running expenses and how it distributes profits.

Unit-linked investments

The scheme members' contributions are used to buy units whose value is linked to an investment fund. The fund's value (and thus that of the units) may rise or fall, depending on the success of the investments. A 'managed' or 'mixed' investment fund usually provides a broad spread of investments.

Deposit-based and with-profits schemes tend to be more secure, whereas unit-linked schemes are more dependent upon stock market performance and are therefore more risky.

The intended time span of an investment can be an important factor influencing choice. Deposit-based schemes are usually more attractive to someone drawing a pension within a few years; it ensures that a possible fall in market prices does not cause difficulties.

However, younger people may prefer a unit-linked scheme, because it can yield a higher return over a long period and short-term fluctuations in the market may not be particularly significant. Of course, it is possible to spread any risk by opting for a mixture of a with-profits scheme and a unit-linked scheme. It is also possible to switch from a unit-linked to a with-profits or deposit-based scheme a year or two before retirement, in order to avoid the risk of a market downturn.

General practitioners

Although GPs are taxed under schedule D as self-employed independent contractors, they are eligible for tax relief on their contributions to the NHS scheme. This is allowed by the Inland Revenue as a concession (known as the A9 concession); it is not a statutory right. This unique arrangement allows GPs to contribute to a PPP whilst remaining members of the NHS scheme and may be done in either of the following ways.

1 By using income not taken into account for NHS scheme purposes, ie 'topping up'

The income available for a PPP is the difference between net relevant earnings (NRE) and NHS superannuable income in any year. Superannuable income is calculated by multiplying the basic 6% NHS scheme contributions by $\frac{100}{6}$. A GP's NRE consist of earned income (both NHS and private) less expenses allowed under schedule D. NRE are subject to the earnings cap, which is currently £78 600 (see Chapter 1).

For example:

Annual contributions paid	£2400
Superannuable income	$£2400 \times \dfrac{100}{6} = £40\,000$
Net relevant earnings (ie schedule D)	£45 000
Income available for PPP	£5000
Allowable premium (depends on age – assume an age of 48)	25% of £5000 = £1250

Therefore £1250 can be used for contributions to a PPP, and these will attract tax relief.

2 Renunciation of tax relief

GPs may choose to forgo tax relief on their basic NHS pension scheme contributions. All NRE can then be used to contribute to a PPP (subject to the earnings cap). In effect, this means that NHS superannuable income is being pensioned twice. Tax relief must also be forgone on any added years or unreduced lump sum being purchased. It is not possible to contribute to AVCs or FSAVCs if tax relief is forgone on basic NHS pension scheme contributions. This is an extremely tax-efficient option, and the pension benefits accruing can be substantial, as can its cost. It is vital that the relative costs and benefits are carefully considered. Under this arrangement, outgoings will form a higher percentage of income; a choice has to be made as to the extent to which today's standard of living should be sacrificed for future retirement benefits.

The following example illustrates the point.

Cost of NHS pension scheme

6% of £40 000 (superannuable income)	£2400
less tax relief (at 40%)	£960
Cost	£1440

Cost of forgoing tax relief and paying maximum contributions into a PPP

6% of £40 000 (superannuable income, no tax relief)	£2400
plus cost of PPP:	
25% of £45 000 (NRE):	£11 250
less tax relief (40%)	£4500
	£6750
Total cost	£9150

Summary of cost of these two alternatives:

NHS pension scheme	£1440
Forgoing tax relief	£9150
Additional cost	£7710

Spouses' pension schemes

It can be extremely advantageous to a GP to contribute towards a PPP for a spouse employed by the practice. If the spouse's salary is just below the limit at which national insurance becomes payable (approximately £2900 per annum in 1994/95), no tax or national insurance is payable on this income, by either the GP (for whom it is a legitimate business expense) or the spouse.

By buying a PPP for the spouse in respect of this income, the GP can also claim tax relief at the usual 40% rate. The investment fund accrued is tax free (as for all PPPs), and 25% of it can be taken as a tax-free lump sum at retirement. The balance must be drawn as pension, although if a spouse has no other income, this is usually tax free. It can be seen that the overall result is an exceptionally tax-efficient form of investment.

The Inland Revenue introduced restrictions on these arrangements from 1 September 1994. Schemes starting after that date are subject to a much lower annual contribution level; there is a transitional arrangement for existing schemes, which defers the implementation of these new limits until 1 September 1999.

Carry-forward of unused tax relief and carry-back of contributions

Tax relief on PPPs is given in the tax year in which the contribution is paid. Unused tax relief can be carried forward for up to six tax years and used in the current tax year.

The carry-back provision may also be used. This enables an individual to elect to have a contribution treated as having been paid in the preceding year or, if there were no net relevant earnings in that preceding year, in the tax year before that.

7

Financial planning for retirement: investments
other than pensions   JOHN WINN

> Why use non-pension investments? • General principles
> • Types of savings and investment schemes • The costs of
> investment • Capital gains tax (CGT)

The tax efficiency of using the wide variety of pension-based facilities make these the first choice for most NHS staff wishing to provide for their retirement. However, there are a wide range of non-pension-based savings and investment schemes that can be used as part of the retirement planning process.

Why use non-pension investments?

There are three main reasons why non-pension-based investments might be appropriate.

1 *Flexibility.* Savings and investment schemes can provide capital or income, or sometimes both, at a time that fits one's plans, rather than at a predetermined date, ie the age of 60. They can also be encashed earlier than intended if circumstances change.

2 *No investment limits.* Unlike pension-based plans, where only a maximum percentage of the appropriate income can be contributed, other investment schemes are only limited to what can sensibly be afforded.
   Payments can be made on a regular basis from disposable income or lump sums, perhaps arising from an unexpected inheritance, can be invested.

3 *Risk versus reward.* If one has a strong base of pension provision, one may wish to invest in areas such as shares, where the potential rewards are high but where there can be short-term risks. However, the advantages and disadvantages of such investments must be understood

and accepted. One simple piece of advice is that if the thought of an investment with 'risks' keeps you awake at night, *do not* invest in such a plan.

The range of non-pension-based schemes is enormous, and this chapter will concentrate on those most commonly available.

To start, there are some general comments that apply to all investment schemes and which need to be recognized in your own financial plan.

General principles

Inflation

Any positive rate of inflation will erode the value of savings and investments. For example, £1000 under the mattress for five years when inflation is running at 5% per annum, will at the end of that time be worth, in real terms, £774. If the £1000 were invested, obtaining 7% interest per annum net of tax, then, using the same inflation figure, the money, in real terms, would be worth approximately £1085.

Taxation

Most savings and investment vehicles will give rise to some form of potential tax liability, either income tax or capital gains tax, or sometimes both. There are some exceptions, and these are described in more detail later in this chapter.

However, the sensible use of independent taxation for a spouse can alleviate some of the potential liability. For example, a man inherits £10 000 and wishes to save this in a building society. He pays tax at 40% on his income, but his wife, who has no earned income, does not pay tax. It would therefore be better for the money to be invested in the wife's name – the building society can be told of the 'non-taxable' status and pay the interest gross.

Early encashment

A good financial plan should contain the flexibility to meet changing circumstances. However, a dramatic change might mean encashing investments earlier than envisaged. Whilst the majority of the most widely used schemes allow this, there could be encashment 'penalties', such as a loss of interest or a predetermined charge.

Security

There are hundreds of institutions willing to look after one's hard earned money. They range from banks and building societies, through government-backed schemes, such as National Savings, to insurance companies, unit trust and investment trust managers. Investment should be with those institutions who can demonstrate the appropriate financial strength, even if this means taking a slightly lower return.

In some instances, there will be compensation schemes in force, for example, bank deposits, investment in insurance companies through the Policyholders Protection Act and the Investors Compensation Scheme. However, these are limited in their scope.

Having considered some generalities, let us now look at the various types of savings and investment schemes available. The following are compiled broadly on the basis of risk, so, for example, deposit accounts, where the capital is secure, are low risk and come first. At the other end are investment trusts, in which the value of the investment depends upon the value of the shares in which the trusts themselves invest. Most of the schemes described will accept regular monthly investment or lump sums. However, some of the National Savings products and the guaranteed bonds issued by insurance companies are only available for lump sum investment.

Types of savings and investment schemes

Deposit accounts

These accounts are operated by banks, building societies and a small number of other financial institutions. In broad terms, money is deposited with the institution and they agree to pay a certain rate of interest, depending upon the facilities required and the period that they keep the money.

The lowest rates of interest are usually paid for 'instant access' accounts where, as the name implies, money can be withdrawn at any time and without notice. If one is prepared to give notice of withdrawal, typically 30 or 90 days, the interest rate will be higher. However, for the best rates the money must be committed for longer periods, typically between one and five years.

If an instant access or short notice account is chosen, one must keep a close watch on the rates of interest paid. Some building societies have, in the past, closed certain accounts, reduced the interest payable and not advised depositors of this situation.

Unless a person registers as a non-taxpayer, the bank or building society will deduct basic rate tax from the interest payable. If one pays higher rate tax, there will be an additional liability for the difference between basic and higher rate, which will be collected through the annual assessment.

Tax Exempt Special Savings Accounts (TESSAs)

These are operated by banks and building societies. Each person is allowed to save in one TESSA and, providing the capital remains in the account for five years, all interest received will be tax free. Savings can either be made monthly, up to a maximum of £150 per month, or by lump sum payments as follows:

Year 1	£3000
Year 2	£1800
Year 3	£1800
Year 4	£1800
Year 5	£600

The maximum savings over five years is £9000. Interest can be withdrawn during the period and will be subject to income tax at the time. If the capital remains intact for the full period, the tax paid on the interest is refunded.

Some institutions operate 'money market' accounts, which pay interest according to the short-term rates available in the market place. Interest from these accounts tends to be better than from the instant access accounts but lower than from the notice and fixed period deposits.

For the taxpayer, there are a small number of offshore deposit accounts. These are usually run by substantial institutions and operate in 'tax havens', such as Jersey. The interest rates will be dictated by the notice period, but interest is paid gross. If the account allows the interest to be 'rolled up', tax is only due when the interest is brought back into the UK.

National Savings

The government operates a range of products through the National Savings organization, full details of which are available from Post Offices.

The National Savings Bank operates two deposit accounts. For the ordinary account, the first £70 of interest is exempt from tax, whereas for the investment account, which pays interest gross, there is a full tax liability at the individual's highest personal rate. Interest rates, particularly for the ordinary account, are not particularly competitive.

More attractive rates are available for the longer-term products. At the time of writing, the first option bond offers a rate guaranteed for 12 months. At the end of this period, the investment can be retained, if the rate for the next 12 months is attractive, or encashed. Basic rate tax is deducted at source, and higher rate taxpayers will have an additional liability.

A similar product, the capital bond, operates over a five-year period. However, its interest is credited gross, so taxpayers at all levels have a liability. For taxpayers, particularly those paying higher rate tax, the savings certificates and index-linked certificates may be more attractive. These again operate over five years, with guaranteed rates. However, the rates are free of all income tax and capital gains tax liability.

Savings certificates pay a known, fixed rate over the period. The index-linked issues pay a fixed rate in addition to the rise in the retail prices index over the five years.

For those wishing to invest smaller monthly amounts, the recently withdrawn National Savings Yearly Plan and Save-as-You-Earn scheme have provided reasonable returns. If the longer-term plans need to be encashed early the capital is normally repaid intact, but there may be reductions in the interest rate.

One word of warning: issues of the yearly plan or savings certificates, including the index-linked version, that have matured should not be left on the general extension rate, where the interest is usually very low.

Government stock (gilts)

Governments issue stock to finance their expenditure, and this can be bought and sold through the National Savings Stock Register. Details are available from most Post Offices. Dividends are paid gross but are liable to income tax, although the sale proceeds are not liable to capital gains tax. However, the price paid will depend upon supply and demand.

For example, a gilt with a high coupon, that is the dividend paid, is likely to command a higher purchase price than a low coupon gilt. The following example should illustrate this. At the time of writing, the stock called Treasury 13.5% 2004–2008 was being valued at £128. This stock promises to repay £100 sometime between 2004 and 2008, the date to be decided by the government. However, in the meantime, income of £13.50 will be paid each year, making a very attractive return of approximately 10.5% gross, even allowing for the higher value. However, if the holder wishes to encash the stock prior to redemption, the value will be that available on the market, which could be higher or lower than the price paid.

Friendly societies

Registered friendly societies are exempt from corporation tax in respect of certain investment plans. In broad terms, the proceeds from a plan that runs for 10 years will be paid without any tax liability, even for higher rate taxpayers. However, because of this tax status, the amount that can be invested is limited to a maximum of £18 per month for each individual.

Guaranteed bonds

From time to time, the internal tax position for some insurance companies will allow them to issue fixed-rate, guaranteed bonds. These are usually for periods of between one and five years. The interest can be 'rolled up' to provide a capital sum at the end of the period. However, interest is credited net of basic rate tax, which cannot be reclaimed by the non-taxpayer. A higher rate taxpayer will have an additional liability.

Collective investments

In simple terms, a collective investment is where a number of individual investors with similar objectives group together, usually under the auspices of a professional investment manager, to pool their resources. Each individual investor shares in the pool in ratio to the money invested and the subsequent value of the assets of the pool. The two most widely used collective investments are investment bonds, operated by insurance companies, and unit trusts, run by many financial institutions.

Investment bonds

Life assurance companies introduced investment bonds as an alternative to unit trusts, although the tax structure is different. The investor buys units in a chosen fund for which the investment objective meets the investor's aims. There is a wide range of funds, from those that invest in cash and fixed-interest stock to pure equity investments in most of the world's stockmarkets. However, many investors look for a broad spread of investment types within their chosen fund to lower the risk. Three types of fund are used by a majority of investors, these being the managed or mixed fund, the with-profits fund and the distribution fund.

The managed fund contains a broad spread of equities, both UK and international, cash, fixed interest and, in many cases, property. This mixture tends to even out the peaks and troughs of investment cycles.

The with-profits fund has gained popularity in the last two or three years. Here, the insurance company adds 'interest' or 'bonuses' to the investment, which, whilst arising from the underlying assets like equities, are smoothed out into a reasonably regular pattern. However, like all such investments, the growth is not guaranteed, and the managers reserve the right to penalize early withdrawal in certain circumstances.

The distribution fund tends to be a cautious mixture of investment types, designed to give steady growth or income as required.

All investment bond funds are liable to capital gains and corporation tax on their internal movements. However, the companies manage their affairs in such a way as largely to avoid capital gains tax. The reserve to meet this liability is usually in the order of 10–15%, which is reflected in the unit price.

Similarly, withdrawals of either regular amounts or irregular lump sums can be used to provide income on a tax-deferred basis. Up to 5% of the original investment can be withdrawn each year with no immediate tax charge. Withdrawals greater than 5% only attract a liability if the holder is a higher rate taxpayer at the time of the withdrawal. This can be used to good effect where, for example, the investment is made prior to retirement. In many cases, the investor will be a higher rate taxpayer at this stage. However, if income reduces after retirement and falls below the higher rate tax threshold, the income can be taken from the bond with no further tax liability, unless this extra income takes the level back over the threshold again.

For those with the ability to plan 10 years prior to retirement, the funds associated with investment bonds can be accessed by regular monthly payments. These plans are known as maximum investment plans.

Unit trusts

Unit trusts provide the investor with a simple doorway to the stockmarkets of the world through professional fund management groups. However, unlike investment bonds, unit trusts invest in stocks and shares, and sometimes cash, but not in areas such as property. Bearing this in mind, unit trusts tend to be more volatile than some of the investment bonds but can give higher returns over a long period.

The managers bear no tax on their dealings with the trusts. Therefore, the individual investor has an income tax liability on dividends, even if these are reinvested within the trust. In addition, disposals of all or part of the investment will give rise to a capital gains tax liability.

However, within the unit trust field, investors can find some relief from tax by investing in a Personal Equity Plan (PEP). These plans, when operated by a recognized PEP manager, attract no income tax or capital gains tax and need not even be declared on a tax return.

At the time of writing, each individual can invest up to £6000 in unit or investment trusts plus a further £3000 in a single share PEP. However, only one PEP can be purchased in each tax year.

With the advent of wider trading within the EEC, more collective investment schemes are being offered from offshore bases such as Luxembourg, Dublin and the Channel Islands. Many of these schemes are operated by substantial UK-based institutions and can often be worthy of serious consideration.

Investment trusts

An investment trust is a limited company that buys and sells shares. As for a unit trust, investors are pooled together, but, unlike a unit trust, the managers can borrow money to increase their investment capability. This is called 'gearing' and can provide higher growth when stockmarkets are rising. Conversely, it can also be the cause of a greater drop in price when markets are falling.

Investment trusts can also be more complex than unit trusts, by the manager creating shares that only reflect the capital growth in the company and ones that receive all the dividend income. Investors must fully understand the impact of such split shares and not think they all have the same characteristics.

As with unit trusts, there are a large number of different trusts available, and care must be taken to select one that fits the individual's risk profile. It must also be remembered that investment in overseas stockmarkets bring the added exposure to currency movements, which can have a major impact on unit prices.

Buying shares

Of all the investment vehicles so far described, this is the one that brings the most risk for the individual. Most private investors have only a limited amount of capital that should be exposed to the risk of the stockmarket. This capital is not usually sufficient to buy a range of shares in sufficient quantity to spread the risk of one share going wrong. For example, £1000 may buy a few shares in Marks and Spencers, whereas a good UK unit trust will provide a stake in 40 to 50 companies for the same price.

Shares can be bought through a stockbroker. Many of the big city firms do not deal with private individuals unless they have £50 000 or more to invest. However, there are some excellent provincial stockbrokers who will deal at much lower amounts. In addition, there are one or two large institutions who have established direct dealings desks for share buyers. These desks will not give advice but will buy or sell on a client's instructions.

The costs of investment

Many of the investment vehicles described here have no discernible costs associated with them. For example, a building society does not charge for opening an account. However, in this case, one is paying for the service in terms of a lower interest rate. On the other hand, investment bonds and units trusts have very clear charging structures, both initial and annual, so the purchaser knows the full costs involved and is given the full benefit of the growth that the investment makes.

Remember, you do not get something for nothing.

Capital gains tax (CGT)

Reference has been made at various points in this chapter to capital gains tax (CGT). Currently, certain investments attract potential CGT on profits, after allowing for inflation, that are in excess of the allowance given to each individual, which is at present £5800.

So, for example, let us assume you invested £10 000 in a unit trust and sold it for £20 000 after 10 years. During that 10 years, inflation had been a total of 25%. Therefore, the original investment of £10 000 is deemed to be revalued at £12 500 (£10 000 + 25%), so the real profit is £7500. From this will be taken the allowance of £5800, leaving a taxable gain of £1700. If you are paying 40% tax at the time, your CGT liability is £680 – not too high a price to pay for good growth.

This chapter has only been able to touch upon some of the most widely used investment plans. It has not been able to go into too much detail and cannot touch on the more esoteric investments, such as antiques and fine wines.

Each individual will have his or her own view, and investment plans must encompass these. To achieve a good plan and keep it running to meet one's changing needs, one must seek advice. A good independent financial adviser will act as a guide through the minefield of investment and ensure there is no sleep lost.

Finally, remember the old saying 'If something looks too good to be true – it probably is'. Sensible investments should give good returns over reasonable time periods, rather than turning the investor into a millionaire, or losing all his or her money overnight.

8

The NHS pension scheme: insurance and family benefits

Ill-health retirement • Death in service • Death after retirement • Death after leaving the scheme but before pensionable age • Additional widower's pension • Remarriage • Divorce • Judicial separation • Allocation • NHS injury benefits scheme

Ill-health retirement

A scheme member who has to retire on the grounds of ill health is usually eligible for an enhanced pension and lump sum. Ill-health retirement has to be approved by the NHS pensions agency and is only applicable to scheme members with at least two years' service who are permanently incapable of carrying out their NHS duties as a result of an illness of body or mind.

Scheme members seeking retirement on ill-health grounds should apply on a form that is available from employers, FHSAs and Health Boards. The completed form must include a medical report, normally from the member's own GP and/or consultant, but medical reports and evidence from other verifiable sources may be taken into account. *Permanent* incapacity must be established. The responsibility for advising the scheme on medical matters rests solely with its medical advisers, and the final decision rests with the NHS pension agencies (see Appendix A). If ill-health retirement is approved, the pension and lump sum benefits should then be applied for on the usual form for normal retirement.

Once ill-health retirement has been approved by the agency, the approval remains valid for one year. If retirement has not taken place within that year, a new application for ill-health retirement needs to be made.

Box 8.1   Ill-health retirement valid for a year

Dr L was suffering from severe depression and, after a great deal of heart-searching, eventually decided to apply for ill-health retirement. This application was successful, but the doctor then decided that she wanted to attempt to continue working, in the hope that this would help her to get better. She wrote to the pensions agency and withdrew her ill-health retirement, and this withdrawal was accepted. Unfortunately, her condition deteriorated and soon after she needed to stop work but was concerned that she would have to go through the full process of an ill-health retirement application all over again. In fact, this proved to be unnecessary because an ill-health retirement approval is valid for 12 months.

From the BMA's files

Enhancing length of service

A member retiring on the grounds of ill health receives an enhanced pension and lump sum, depending upon length of service and age. Service cannot be enhanced beyond 40 years in total (including any added years being purchased). In most cases, service can also not be enhanced beyond what would have been achieved at the age of 60. However, enhancement to the age of 65 is permitted in cases where service has been less than 20 years (which provides an extra insurance element for older members with relatively short service) (Table 8.1).

Table 8.1   Enhancement of service on ill-health retirement

Length of service (years)	Enhancement (years)
Less than 5	Nil
5–10	Doubled (limit age 65)
10–20	Increased to 20 (limit age 65)
	or, if better
	$6\frac{2}{3}$ (limit age 60)
20+	$6\frac{2}{3}$ (limit age 60)

For example, a 54-year-old with 30 years' service has the following:

- a potential maximum enhancement of $6\frac{2}{3}$ years
- a limitation of years to the age of 60
- an actual enhancement therefore of 6 years.

What benefits are paid on ill-health retirement?

The enhanced pension and lump sum will be based on the enhanced service shown in Table 8.1. For service of less than two years, a refund of contributions is paid (or a non-enhanced pension and lump sum if over the age of 60). For service of between two and five years, a pension and lump sum are paid, but these are not enhanced.

Calculating the benefits

The first step is to calculate pension accrued to date (see Chapter 2 for non-practitioners and Chapter 3 for practitioners). This accrued pension is then enhanced by the amount shown in Table 8.1 The example below shows how this applies to someone retiring on ill-health grounds at the age of 54, with 30 years' previous service and an accrued pension of £17 000:

Previous service to date	30 years
Service enhancement	6 years (limit age 60)
Total	36 years
Enhancement factor	$\dfrac{36}{30}$
Accrued pension to date	£17 000
Ill-health pension	£17 000 × $\dfrac{36}{30}$ = £20 400

In this case the pension has been enhanced by £3400 per annum (£20 400 − £17 000). The lump sum enhancement is three times the pension enhancement, ie £10 200.

Added years

There is an important insurance element underlying the purchase of added years; if a member retires on the grounds of ill health, full credit is given for the added years being bought, even though the contract to purchase them has not been completed. The only exceptions are:

- if the ill-health retirement is on or after age 60
- if the ill-health retirement is applied for less than 12 months after starting to purchase added years.

If the member is subsequently re-employed in the NHS and rejoins the scheme, contributions due under the added years contract again become payable, even though full credit has already been given.

Re-employment in the NHS

Ill-health retirement does not prevent someone from being re-employed in the NHS, providing it is in a different or reduced capacity. Prior to 6 March 1995, it was possible to rejoin the NHS pension scheme; since then, only someone re-employed in the NHS before the age of 50 can rejoin the scheme.

Members who have left the NHS

An ill-health pension can be paid to scheme members whose ill health occurs after leaving the NHS if their health problems mean that they are incapable of undertaking any regular employment. However, their accrued service is not enhanced unless it can be shown retrospectively that ill-health retirement would have been appropriate when they left the NHS.

Illness or injury caused by NHS duties

In these circumstances, injury benefit may be paid; details of the NHS injury benefits scheme are provided below.

Practitioners holding other posts

It is possible that a medical condition may justify ill-health retirement from practitioner work but allow non-practitioner work to continue (and vice versa).

Terminal ill health

From 6 March 1995, in cases where life expectancy is less than 12 months, the ill-health pension can be commuted into a tax-free amount of five times that pension, subject to an overriding cap equal to two times pay minus the retirement lump sum. The retirement lump sum, usually three times the pension, is payable in addition to the commuted amount. There will be no reduction in either figure in respect of pre-1972 service. However, the commuted amount will be reduced by the amount of guaranteed minimum pension payable: this is non-commutable and is that element of the NHS pension that must be paid under State pension legislation. Dependants' benefits will still be payable as usual.

Death in service

Life assurance: the death gratuity

Insurance cover is provided immediately upon joining the NHS pension scheme; a tax-free lump sum (known as the death gratuity) is paid if a scheme member dies in service. Since 6 March 1995, this gratuity has been twice annual salary; for practitioners, this means that it is twice the average annual dynamized remuneration. No deduction will be made in respect of pre-1972 service (which, as explained earlier, usually resulted in a reduced lump sum). Prior to 6 March 1995, the amount of the death gratuity was the highest of the following options:

- three times the pension the member would have received if retiring on grounds of ill health at the date of death (see example above) less any deduction in respect of pre-1972 service

- one year's pensionable salary based on the best of the last three years

- a refund of the member's contributions with compound interest at $2\frac{1}{2}\%$ per annum.

For members with less than one year's service in the scheme, the gratuity was the equivalent of one year's salary.

The death gratuity is normally paid directly to the member's spouse. Anyone who wishes to opt out of this arrangement should complete a special form (available from employers, FHSAs and Health Boards) and send it to the NHS pensions agency. If this option applies or the member does not have a spouse, the gratuity is paid into the member's estate and is therefore liable for assessment for inheritance tax.

Widow's/widower's pensions

An enhanced pension will usually be paid to widows or widowers of members with at least five years in the scheme.

- *Widow's pension*: half the ill-health pension that would have been paid at the date of death (see example above).

- *Widower's pension*: the same as the widow's pension but based on service since 6 April 1988 only (for exceptions, see 'Additional widower's pension' on page 81).

These benefits are paid three months after the member's death. During this interim period, a short-term pension is paid, which is equal to the actual rate of the member's pensionable salary at date of death. If there are dependent children, this three-month, short-term pension is extended to six months.

For service of between two and five years, the same short-term pension is paid, but there is no enhancement of any subsequent widow's or widower's pension (because, as explained above, these pensions are based on ill-health pensions, which are not enhanced if service is less than 5 years).

For service of less than two years, the short-term pension is paid for the first three (or six) months, but no pension is paid thereafter (unless the member was aged 60 or over). However, a pension may be paid in respect of this service under the SERPs arrangements (see Chapter 17).

Box 8.2   Sad consequences of a job change

Dr C was 50 years of age and had been in the Universities Superannuation Scheme (USS) for 25 years. He took up an NHS post and joined the NHS scheme, leaving his USS benefits in the USS. Sadly, he died suddenly within a few months of joining the NHS, with unfortunate and unforeseen financial consequences for his wife and two children:

- had he stayed at the university, the widow's pension would have been based on service enhanced to the age of 65 (an extra 15 years). Because he had left, the service was not enhanced at all

- the same problem arose with the children's allowance (see below)

- because NHS service was less than two years, an NHS widow's pension was only payable for six months.

From the BMA's files

Child allowance

The amount of child allowance paid is based on the enhanced pension that would have been paid had the member retired on the grounds of ill health at the date of death, except that if the member's service had been less than five years, this is increased to 10 years (or to that amount of service which would have been accrued by the age of 65 if this is less than 10 years).

If a widow's/widower's pension is being paid, one quarter of the enhanced pension is paid as child allowance (one half if there are two or more children). The maximum total of survivors' pensions paid in these circumstances is therefore half to the spouse and half to the children, ie 100% of the member's enhanced pension.

In cases where no widow's/widower's pension is being paid, one-third of the enhanced pension is paid as child allowance, two-thirds being paid if there are two or more children.

During the period that a short-term pension is being paid to a widow or widower (see above), no child allowance is payable. However, if no widow's/widower's pension is payable, the child allowance is paid immediately, at the deceased member's rate of salary for 6 months and thereafter at the usual rate of one-third of the enhanced pension.

Box 8.3 Help for orphaned children

Two doctors, husband and wife, died in a car accident overseas, leaving two dependent children at school in England.

A year later, the children's guardian approached the BMA for help because no benefits had been paid. Enquiries showed that this delay resulted from a bizarre sequence of misunderstandings and bureaucratic muddles.

In fact, one doctor was a member of the NHS pension scheme and the other a member of the Civil Service pension scheme, and after further protracted struggle it was possible to obtain for the children:

- a child allowance at the one-third rate for each child from both pension schemes

- a death gratuity from both pension schemes

- an ex gratia payment by way of compensation for the long delay.

From the BMA's files

Child allowance is payable for any children dependent on the deceased scheme member. It can be paid to anyone who has care of the children, or directly to the children if they look after themselves.

The child is regarded as dependent if under the age of 17, in full-time education or training, or permanently incapable of earning a living as a result of ill health or handicap.

A wide range of children are potentially eligible, including:

- the deceased member's child, grandchild, stepchild or legally adopted child

- a brother, sister, nephew or niece of the member or spouse (including half brothers, etc)

- any child dependent upon the member for two years, or half the child's life if this is less

- a child born within 12 months of the member's death.

Box 8.4 Seven children

Dr E had four children by his first marriage, three of whom were still at university or school, ie dependent. He also had three young stepchildren from his second marriage.

His natural children were effectively provided for in the event of his death by means of insurance policies, and he therefore wanted the NHS child allowance to be paid to his stepchildren only.

Normally, for six dependent children, the child allowance would be split equally between them; there is no provision to assign benefits from one family to another. It also needs to be kept in mind that where there are dependent children with a surviving parent who has no entitlement to a widow's pension (ie Dr E's first wife), the rate of child allowance is higher (the one-third rate rather than the one-quarter).

The pensions agency was unable to give a definitive judgement before the date of death, because at that time each case will be looked at on its merits, with particular attention being paid to whether or not each child is dependent at that time and, if so, to what extent.

From the BMA's files

Added years

Members under the age of 60 who die in service (or within 12 months of leaving service) will receive full credit for any added years being purchased.

AVCs/FSAVCs

If AVC contributors die before retirement, the full accumulated value of the fund is paid by Equitable Life. In addition, an amount is payable by way of life assurance if the member chose to secure this by making AVCs (see Chapter 5 for details). FSAVC schemes may have similar arrangements; the member's dependents should contact the FSAVC provider for details.

Death after retirement

Life assurance: the death gratuity

A lump sum death gratuity may be payable if death occurs within five years of retirement. Since 6 March 1995, this is equivalent to five years' pension, subject to an overriding maximum figure of twice the annual salary at retirement less the lump sum paid at retirement.

Widow's/widower's pensions

Marriage before retirement
For the first three months after the death (six months if there are dependent children), the widow's/widower's pension is paid at the same rate as the pension being paid at the date of death. Thereafter the amount paid is as follows:

- Widow's pension: half of the member's pension

- Widower's pension: as for widows, but based on service since 6 April 1988 only (for exceptions, see 'Additional widower's pension' below).

Marriage after retirement

- Widow's pension: half of the member's pension, but based on service since 6 April 1978 only

- Widower's pension: half of the member's pension, but based on service since 6 April 1988 only (for exceptions, see below).

Child allowance

The child allowance is based on the member's actual pension at date of death, except that service of less than 10 years will be increased to 10 years (subject to the usual limit of 65 years of age). The proportion of member's pension payable as child allowance is described above in the section on 'Death in service'.

If a widow's/widower's pension is payable, no child allowance is paid for the first six months after the member's death. If no widow's/widower's pension is payable, the child allowance is paid immediately, for six months at the rate of the deceased member's pension and thereafter at the usual rate.

The child allowance is paid to any child who is dependent upon the member at both retirement and date of death.

Death after leaving the scheme but before pensionable age

Life assurance: the death gratuity

A death gratuity is payable, which is normally three times the pension the member would have received at the date of death. This is reduced if the normal lump sum payable under the scheme would have been less than three times the pension (see Chapter 2).

Widow's/widower's pensions

Marriage before leaving the scheme

- If death occurs within 12 months of leaving the scheme, the widow's/ widower's pension is calculated as for death in service. In most cases, this provides an enhanced pension.

- If death occurs more than 12 months after leaving the scheme, the widow's pension is based on one half of the member's accrued pension and the widower's pension is based on one half of the member's accrued pension since 6 April 1988. Thus, there is no enhancement of pension.

In both cases the pension starts at the date of death (there being no special short-term pension paid for the first three months as for death in service).

Marriage after leaving the scheme
In these circumstances there is no enhancement of pension; the widow's pension is based on service since 6 April 1978 and the widower's pension on service since 6 April 1988.

Child allowance

The child allowance is based on the pension a member would have received had he or she retired at date of death, except that service of less than 10 years is increased to 10 years (subject again to the usual limit of age 65). The proportion of the member's pension payable as child allowance is the same as that described above in the section on death in service. The child allowance commences from the day after the date of death.

The child allowance is paid to any child dependent on the member upon leaving the scheme and at the date of death.

Additional widower's pension

The widower's pension is normally paid only in respect of the member's service since 6 April 1988. However, there are exceptional circumstances in which a full widower's pension is paid, which include:

- where a female member opted to buy a widower's pension in respect of pre-1988 service

- where a female member's husband is dependent as a result of permanent illness and a nomination has been accepted by the scheme.

Chapter 2 provides details of these arrangements.

Box 8.5 Helping a family left behind

A young woman doctor was diagnosed as having terminal cancer and was concerned that the pension payable to her husband and two young children would be based on service since 1988 only.

First, we were able to assure her that the post-1988 restriction does not apply to the child allowance and that both children would receive the full child allowance until the age of 17, or beyond that age if they were still in full-time education.

However, the doctor also mentioned that she was concerned about her husband's pension because he would have no other income. It transpired that this was because he had a physical disability that prevented him from earning a living. Because of these circumstances, the doctor was able, before she died, to nominate her husband for full widower's pension on all her service.

From the BMA's files

Remarriage

The widow's/widower's pension will be withdrawn on remarriage (or if living together as man and wife) unless financial hardship can be proved. It may be restored if the second marriage or relationship comes to an end.

Box 8.6   Widow's pension withdrawn on remarriage

Mrs H was 45 when her GP husband died. Although an NHS widow's pension is not reduced if extra income is obtained from taking a job, Mrs H was not able to work because of a long-term illness. After a time, she received an offer of marriage from someone who was not wealthy but who had a steady income. The pensions agency's view was that withdrawing the pension on remarriage in this case would not have caused 'severe financial hardship', and Mrs H was therefore forced to choose between remarriage and her widow's pension.

From the BMA's files

Divorce

No widow's or widower's pension is payable to a divorced partner (see Chapter 18).

Judicial separation

For those who retire after 6 March 1995, a judicial separation will not affect the payment of a widow's/widower's pension. The pension will be payable provided that the couple are not divorced.

The position is different in respect of scheme members who retired before 6 March 1995, even if they die after that date. In this case, the widow's pension is payable in full only if there is an order for maintenance at the date of death. If there is no such order, the widow's pension is payable on service since 6 April 1978 only.

In any case, the widower's pension is payable only on service since 6 April 1988.

Box 8.7   78 years young

Dr B is 78 years of age and he retired in 1982. He has lived with his current partner (Jane) for 10 years, having had a child (Stephen) with her. Dr B and Jane have not married because he has not divorced his wife (Rebecca). He was concerned about what would happen if he died. The answer was:

- Jane would get no pension unless Dr B divorced Rebecca and married Jane. Even then, the pension would only be based on his service since 6 April 1978, ie only four years, as he retired in 1982

- Rebecca would not receive a pension if they divorced. If the divorce did not go through before he died, she would receive a full widow's pension (because following their judicial separation he was paying support as a result of a court order)

- Stephen would receive nothing because he was not dependent upon Dr B when he retired (not having been born at that stage!)

- the death gratuity would be paid into Dr B's estate and would go to Jane, because his will specified this (he had completed the necessary form advising the Pensions Agency that he did not want the death gratuity to go to his legal wife).

From the BMA's files

Allocation

Scheme members may give up some of their pension to their spouses or anyone who is partially dependent upon them. The 'allocated pension' is paid in addition to any widow's/widower's pension that may be due.

Up to one-third of the member's pension can be allocated in this way. The size of the recipient's pension depends upon his or her age and sex, the date the allocation is made and the amount of pension given up.

All allocation can be made at or within one month after retirement, after the age of 60 if the scheme member has 40 years' service, or after the age of 65. It cannot be cancelled. If the chosen recipient dies first, the pension cannot be restored to the member. Before allocation, the member must have a medical examination to establish that he or she has a normal life expectancy.

NHS injury benefits scheme

The NHS injury benefits scheme is designed to provide benefits to anyone who suffers injury, illness or disease (referred to here as 'injury') as a result of their NHS duties.

Who is covered by the scheme?

- Everyone employed in the NHS is covered. GPs and honorary contract holders are also covered, but those employed by agencies are not.

- There is no waiting period for eligibility. Cover is provided from the first day of work in the NHS.

- NHS pension scheme membership is not necessary. Members and non-members alike are covered by the injury benefits scheme. The scheme is, however, administered by the pensions agencies.

Where must the injury have occurred?

The injury must be primarily attributable to the person's NHS employment or work and must have occurred:

- while at work
- while a volunteer at an accident or emergency providing assistance required by their professional training and codes of conduct
- off duty but in the general area of work
- off duty but assaulted in connection with NHS duties
- while travelling to or from work with the employer's permission in a vehicle provided or arranged by the employer
- to a GP or district nurse travelling to or in a patient's home
- as part of a hospital call-out team
- in the course of work-related travel.

   The following are not covered:

- journeys to and from work (other than those referred to above)
- injuries resulting mainly from self-negligence or misconduct.

Under what circumstances are benefits payable?

Benefits are payable if:

- the person is temporarily off work without pay or on reduced pay (for example, if the member is on half-pay sick leave)
- the person continues working in the NHS but earnings ability has been permanently reduced by 11% or more
- it is necessary to give up NHS work as a result of the injury
- NHS work finishes for some other reason but the injury has resulted in earning ability being reduced by 11% or more
- the person dies as a result of the injury.

What benefits are payable?

Temporary injury allowance
There is a guaranteed income of 85% of pay.

Permanent injury allowance
Table 8.2 provides details. It shows that benefits involve a guaranteed income as a percentage of pay. The concepts of 'guaranteed income' and 'pay' warrant closer attention.

Table 8.2   Guaranteed income

Reduction of earnings ability	Percentage of pay obtained for years of service				Lump sum
	Less than 5	5–14	15–24	25+	
11–25%	15	30	45	60	12.5
26–50%	40	50	60	70	25.0
51–75%	65	70	75	80	37.5
76% or more	85	85	85	85	50.0

What does 'guaranteed income' consist of?

The injury benefit is actually a balancing figure, or a topping-up of other benefits that may be payable. These benefits are the NHS ill-health retirement pension (and lump sum – see below) and State social security benefits. Thus the guaranteed income comprises the following:

NHS pension
+
State benefits
+
Injury benefits
=
Guaranteed income

For example, if the person is eligible for injury benefits at the rate of 85% of pay, the NHS pension entitlement is 40% of pay and State benefits amount to 20% of pay, the guaranteed income figure consists of the following:

	Pay
NHS pension	40%
State benefits	20%
Injury benefits	25%
Guaranteed income	85%

The injury benefit element is therefore, in this case, a topping-up of 25% of pay.

The injury benefit element, like the NHS ill-health pension, is increased in line with the retail prices index from the date payment commences.

What is 'pay' for the purposes of injury benefit?

As in the NHS pension scheme, pay is deemed to be the earnings received in the best of the last three years of service.

However, unlike the NHS pension scheme, pay consists of actual earnings. The notional whole-time equivalent salary is not used for injury benefit purposes. For part-time staff, this could mean that the NHS pension alone will produce a higher benefit than that payable under the injury benefit scheme, ie an NHS pension of 50% of whole-time salary may result in a higher figure than an injury benefit guaranteed income of 85% of a part-time salary.

For GPs, the pay figure used is the annual average of dynamized superannuable income. This means that the injury benefit (assuming for illustrative purposes that the maximum of 85% is payable) may be more or less than 85% of the GP's current annual income depending upon the circumstances.

- If the GP has recently dropped from full time to part time, perhaps to commence a job share arrangement, the maximum payable will be in excess of 85% of current earnings. This is a valuable insurance benefit for part-time doctors who have previously worked full time.

- On the other hand, GPs who have in recent years started to earn more than earlier in their careers will find that the injury benefit is less than 85% of current annual income.

What is the lump sum payable?

Table 8.2 above shows the amount of lump sum payable as a percentage of pay, depending upon the reduction in earnings ability that the injury has caused.

However, unlike the continuing injury benefit payment, the lump sum is not a topping-up of the NHS pension scheme lump sum. It is paid in addition to this, and it is also entirely tax free.

It follows that injury benefits are always worth applying for, even if only to ensure that the lump sum is obtained.

What State benefits need to be taken into account?

As explained above, certain State benefits need to be taken into account in establishing the guaranteed income figure. These are:

- sickness and invalidity benefit
- industrial disablement benefit.

Other State benefits (eg mobility allowance and attendance allowance) are not taken into account and, if the applicant is eligible, can be paid in addition to the guaranteed income.

Death benefits

If the injury results in death, spouse's and children's benefits are payable, as shown in Table 8.3.

Table 8.3 Death benefits

Dependants	Amount of pay guaranteed following death
Widow/widower only	45%
Each of the first 4 children	10% if there is a widow/widower, or
	20% if there is no widow/widower
Each dependent adult child who is incapacitated	20% if there is a surviving parent, or
	45% if there is no surviving parent
One dependent parent	20% if there is a widow/widower, or
	45% if there is no widow/widower

Taxation

The taxation position of the three elements that make up the guaranteed income can be summarized as follows:

- *NHS pension*: taxable

- *State benefits*: not currently taxable, but under review

- *injury benefits*: temporary injury benefit is taxable, as is permanent injury benefit if the person remains in the same job on reduced earnings. However, permanent injury benefit is not taxable if, as a result of the injury, the person has had to leave the NHS or change jobs within the NHS.

Special arrangements for junior doctors

The NHS scheme makes special arrangements for junior doctors. This takes account of the fact that they would have had the ability to earn a higher income had they gone into general practice at the earliest opportunity. For injury benefit purposes only, their pay is deemed to be a percentage of GP pay. The GP figure used is the average net remuneration figure set each year following the Doctors' and Dentists' Review Body Report.

Table 8.4 shows the specific percentage of GP average net income, which applies to each grade of junior doctor.

Table 8.4 Deemed junior doctor income

Junior doctor grade	Percentage of GP average net remuneration
House officer	53
Senior house officer	65
Registrar	87
Senior registrar	100

An example of the practical effect of these arrangements is given below:

Registrar grade	
Actual salary	£23 325
Deemed injury benefit salary	87% of GP average
87% of £41 890	£36 444
Maximum injury benefit	
85% of £36 444	£30 977

This example shows that the injury benefit payable (£30 977) is significantly in excess of the doctor's actual salary (£23 325) and illustrates the value of this insurance benefit to junior doctors.

Damages and compensation

Separately from the injury benefits scheme, it may be that the injured person is able to pursue a claim for damages or compensation from the employer. This is an area in which specialist legal advice is necessary, and it may be possible to obtain this from a professional association or trade union.

The pensions agency will examine the details of any damages or compensation award, in particular the elements of the award that reflect loss of earnings and/or a reduction in earnings ability, and this may be taken into account in setting the level of injury benefits, possibly leading to a reduction in these benefits. The implications of an award of this kind should be discussed from the outset with a legal adviser and advice sought from the pensions agency.

9

Early retirement

The meaning of the term 'early retirement' varies according to the context in which it is used. The NHS pension scheme has a normal retirement age of 60 years; at the age of 60, NHS scheme members are entitled to retire and receive their pension and lump sum (age 55 for mental health officers/special class status – see Chapter 11). If members retire at age 60 or thereafter, they are said to be taking 'normal retirement'.

If they retire before the age of 60, this is 'early retirement'. The varying circumstances in which early retirement may be taken are summarized in Chapter 10. However, there are also circumstances in which 'early retirement' may occur after the age of 60, namely if a scheme member does not retire normally but retires 'early' before a normal contractual retirement age of 65, often with enhanced benefits.

Retirement in any of the following circumstances, whether before or after the age of 60, is not 'normal retirement':

- redundancy
- organizational change
- in the 'interests of the service'
- 'achieving a balance' arrangements
- under special arrangements for general dental practitioners (GDPs).

Redundancy and organizational change

Early retirement in these circumstances may occur as a result of a reorganization, a reduction in the level of service required or a closure of a unit.

In the interests of the efficiency of the service

These arrangements apply to members who have given valued service in the past but who are no longer able to do so, possibly because of new or expanding duties or a decline in capabilities arising from age or domestic circumstances, or because of health reasons that in themselves are insufficient to warrant ill-health retirement.

'Achieving a balance'

The scheme is intended to release funding to create new consultant posts and applies to consultants and associate specialists aged 50 or over and with at least five years' service. The decision to offer early retirement is at the discretion of the employing authority, which must confirm that:

- the retirement would advance necessary structural changes and be in the interests of the service
- the retiring doctor would be replaced by another consultant.

Partial retirement is also available to whole-time and maximum part-time consultants and associate specialists, aged 60 and over.

The partial retirement arrangement involves splitting the contract into two parts (eg 7/11 and 4/11) and retiring from one of them whilst continuing in the other, thereby enabling doctors to reduce their work-load and claim full NHS pension and lump sum (based on all previous service). There is no provision for enhancement of service and pension in the case of partial retirement.

General dental practitioners (GDPs)

GDPs may volunteer for early retirement with enhanced benefits if they:

- are on the list of an FHSA or Health Board
- are aged 55 or over
- have 10 years' service as a GDP since 1976
- have an appropriate level of superannuable income.

Priority is given to those GDPs who:

- are closest to age 65
- have health problems
- have severe, long-term domestic problems
- have demonstrated a high contribution to general dental services.

Who is eligible for early retirement benefits?

The enhanced benefits associated with early retirement may be paid to a member aged 50 or over with at least five years' service. (Special arrangements apply to GDPs – see above.) For those aged under 50, the benefit is preserved in the NHS pension scheme and paid at normal retirement age; there is no enhancement of service or pension. However a redundancy payment may be payable, as explained below.

Members employed outside the NHS who contribute to the NHS pension scheme under a 'direction facility' (eg some doctors employed by university medical schools) may receive an immediate pension if aged over 50, but this will not necessarily be enhanced (see 'Clinical academic staff' below). The 'direction' arrangements are explained in Chapter 5.

Enhancement of service

Enhanced benefits are based on enhanced service (Table 9.1). Thus a member aged 56 with 30 years' service would be enhanced by nine years

Table 9.1   Enhancement of service

Service	Enhancement
Less than 10 years	Service doubled
10 years or more	10 years

Subject to service not being increased:

- beyond a total of 40 years' calendar service
- beyond age 65

whichever is the less.

(to age 65), whereas a member aged 56 with 36 years' service could only be enhanced four years (to 40 years' service in total).

Calculating the enhanced early retirement pension and lump sum

The example below shows the amount of pension paid to a consultant aged 56 with 30 years' whole-time service.

Normal pension (see Chapter 2)	$\frac{30}{80} \times £51\,165$	$= £19\,187$
	Lump sum	$= £57\,561$
Service	$= 30$ years	
Enhancement (to age 65)	$= 9$ years	
Total enhanced service	$= 39$ years	
Enhancement factor	$\frac{39}{30}$	
Enhanced pension	$\frac{39}{30} \times £19\,187$	$= £24\,943$
	Lump sum	$= £74\,829$

Enhanced benefits
    Pension = £5756 (£24 943 – £19 187)
    Lump sum = £17 268 (£74 829 – £57 561)

Redundancy payments

A scheme member may be eligible for a redundancy payment if early retirement is due to:

- redundancy
- organizational change.

However, no redundancy payment is made if the early retirement is due to:

- the interests of the service
- 'achieving a balance' changes.

Redundancy payments will be reduced if the enhancement of service as shown in Table 9.1 above exceeds $6\frac{2}{3}$ years (Table 9.2).

Table 9.2 How the redundancy payment is reduced

Enhancement	Reduction in redundancy payment (%)
Up to $6\frac{2}{3}$ years	Nil
7 years	10
8 years	40
9 years	70
10 years	100

For example, if a member is eligible for a redundancy payment of £20 000 and his or her service is enhanced by eight years, the redundancy payment will be reduced as follows:

Redundancy payment	£20 000
Reduction (40% of £20 000)	£ 8 000
Actual redundancy payment	£12 000

For ease of calculation, both Table 9.2 and this example show complete years of pensionable service enhancement, each additional complete year resulting in a further 30% reduction in the redundancy payment. In fact, the actual calculation is based on the number of days of enhancement.

Each extra day of enhancement would have resulted in the redundancy payment being reduced by $\frac{1}{365} \times 30\%$.

Redundancy payments are calculated as follows ('year' meaning complete year):

Aged 50 and over (enhanced pension payable)

- One and one half weeks' pay for each year of service at age 41 and over

  plus

- one week's pay for each year from age 22 to age 40

subject to an overall maximum of 30 weeks' pay and 20 years' service. After the age of 64, the redundancy payment is reduced by $\frac{1}{12}$ for each additional month of service.

Aged under 50 (no pension payable)

- Aged 22–40: one week's pay for each year of service (maximum 20 years)
- Aged 41 and over: two weeks' pay for each year at age 18 and over (maximum 50 weeks' pay)

  plus

  two weeks' pay for each year at age 41 and over (maximum 16 weeks' pay)
  Overall maximum: 66 weeks' pay.

'Pay' for redundancy purposes means the actual salary being received at the date of redundancy (rather than salary for pension purposes, which allows part-time salaries to be treated as whole time).

Cost to employing authorities

Because the enhanced pension benefits are regarded as compensation, they are paid by the employer (rather than the NHS pension scheme), who must meet the following costs:

- full cost of pension up to normal retirement age (usually the age of 60 but 55 for MHO/special classes)

- the enhanced element of the pension for life, plus the enhanced element of any subsequent dependants' pensions
  (NB the above two costs include the costs of index linking pensions to the retail prices index)

- that part of the tax-free lump sum relating to the enhanced service

- the additional cost caused by paying the lump sum before normal retirement age

- the redundancy payment.

Clinical academic staff

Early retirement on redundancy or organizational grounds

As explained above, there are essentially two elements to the compensation package paid on redundancy. The first is an enhanced pension and lump sum, available only to those aged 50 and over, and the second is the redundancy payment. For clinical academics employed by a university or medical school, there are complications in relation to both elements of the compensation package.

Turning first to the pension and lump sum element of the package, clinical academics may be members of either the NHS pension scheme or the Universities Superannuation Scheme (USS).

Those in the NHS scheme have been able to retain their NHS scheme membership as a result of the 'direction' arrangements (see Chapter 5 for details), even though they are not NHS employees, and it is this employment status that creates difficulties in respect of redundancy. This is because the NHS compensation package, which is based on the early retirement regulations, does not apply to non-NHS employees; thus the pension and lump sum enhancement is not available as a right to clinical academics.

If a clinical academic member of the NHS pension scheme is made redundant, the pensions agency will arrange for the non-enhanced pension and lump sum to be paid and will inform the non-NHS employer how much the enhanced element would have been. The academic employer must then decide whether it will fund this enhancement or offer an alternative redundancy package.

The position of USS members is technically different, although the outcome is often the same or very similar. For USS members, pension and lump sum enhancement may be available under the premature retirement compensation scheme. This allows for enhancement on the same terms as in the NHS (see Table 9.1). However, it only applies if the academic employer is prepared to provide the funding.

The second element of the compensation package is the redundancy payment. The NHS redundancy terms described above do not apply to clinical academics. Their redundancy terms depend upon the policy adopted by each employing institution. Sometimes these redundancy terms have been better than NHS terms. However, in recent experience, they have tended to be worse. An additional problem arises if employing institutions offset redundancy payments against pension enhancements at a level higher than those applicable to NHS staff (see Table 9.2 for NHS staff).

The position of clinical academics in respect of redundancy is both complicated and potentially unsatisfactory, since they may be offered worse redundancy terms than those available to NHS colleagues. Thus any package being offered must be assessed very carefully, and professional advice should be sought; BMA members should seek advice from their local BMA office.

Some doctors hold honorary contracts within the NHS and are employed by a university or medical school. Alternatively, an 'A + B' contract may be held, whereby a doctor is employed by both the university/medical school and the NHS. Under this arrangement, the doctor's university/medical school employment may be at risk if NHS changes bring the NHS contract to an end. Eligibility for pension enhancement and redundancy payments depends upon the nature of the contract, in particular upon who the employer is. The funding source of enhancement may also depend upon what changes have caused the redundancy. Again, this is an area in which advice should be sought from the local BMA office.

Changes in London

London's health services are undergoing substantial changes as a result of the Tomlinson Report and the effects of the NHS internal market. The government established the London Implementation Group to prepare ways of coping with the effects of these changes, and its recommendations have led to:

- a clearing house being established to assist displaced staff in finding alternative employment. Details of displaced staff and vacant posts are sent to the clearing house and, where possible, displaced individuals are matched with the vacant posts

- agreement on procedures for redundancy selection

- employers being issued with guidance on local selection processes for displaced career-grade medical and dental staff

- special arrangements being agreed to enable consultants outside London to volunteer for early retirement on organizational grounds, in order to create vacancies for displaced London consultants.

The BMA's Central Consultants and Specialists Committee's booklet 'How Might the London Changes Affect You?' is available from local BMA offices.

Indexation

The NHS pension paid on early retirement is increased annually in line with the retail prices index. However, anyone taking early retirement before the age of 55 will not have their pension increased until 55, at which point it is increased in line with changes in the retail prices index to take account of the period that has elapsed since retirement.

Taxing lump sum payments

The first £30 000 of any redundancy payment is tax free, and the enhanced element of the NHS pension scheme lump sum is tax free only within this £30 000 limit.

Pay in lieu of notice is taxed unless it is paid as compensation for a breach of the requirement to give notice. In these circumstances, it is tax free up to the £30 000 limit.

The taxation of termination payments is a complex area, and specialist advice should be obtained from the tax inspector or an accountant.

Returning to work after early retirement

Re-employment is not usually allowed unless the early retirement was due to compulsory redundancy; if it occurs within four weeks, it will result in the loss of the redundancy payment. Permanent re-employment after early retirement under 'achieving a balance' is not allowed, although re-employment as a locum may be permitted.

Since 6 March 1995, rejoining the NHS pension scheme is not permissible after retirement benefits have been taken. Prior to 6 March 1995, it was possible to rejoin the scheme, although this option was usually inadvisable if enhanced service had been granted.

Added years and AVCs/FSAVCs

If a pension and lump sum are payable on early retirement, an added years credit will be given based on the amount of the added years contract completed by the date of retirement, less an actuarial reduction to take account of early payment (see Chapter 5).

If a member retires early with an NHS pension, the accumulated value of the AVC/FSAVC fund must be taken.

10

Voluntary early retirement

Actuarial reduction • Voluntary early retirement without
actuarial reduction • Effect on other early retirement
options • Returning to work

With effect from 6 March 1995, members of the NHS pension scheme
can retire voluntarily at any time after reaching the age of 50. As explained
in Chapter 9, the normal retirement age of the scheme is 60, and a
member can always retire and draw a pension from that age onwards.
However, prior to 6 March 1995, it was not possible to retire before the
age of 60 and draw a pension other than in the circumstances listed in
Table 10.1.

Table 10.1 Early retirement options

- Ill-health retirement (Chapter 8)
- Redundancy, organizational change or in the interests of the service
  (Chapter 9)
- 'Achieving a balance' (Chapter 9)
- Members having special class or mental health officer status (Chapter
  11)
- Early retirement for general dental practitioners (Chapter 9)

Actuarial reduction

Under voluntary early retirement arrangements, the pension is normally
reduced actuarially because it is drawn before the normal retirement age
of 60 and is therefore payable over a longer period. This is a common
feature of most occupational pension schemes. The logic is simple: a
scheme member's early retirement should not result on average in
a greater total amount of pension being paid during the member's lifetime

than would have been paid had the member stayed on until the scheme's normal retirement age. The actuarial reduction ensures that voluntary early retirement does not increase the scheme's overall costs and the contributions required to fund it. Thus the amount of pension and lump sum paid on voluntary early retirement comprise the amount accrued at the date of retirement less any actuarial reduction, which is calculated by the Government Actuary's Department. Table 10.2 shows the proportion of accrued pension and lump sum paid on voluntary early retirement from age 50 to 59.

Table 10.2 Proportion of benefit payable

Age	Pension	Lump sum
50	0.599	0.747
51	0.624	0.769
52	0.652	0.792
53	0.682	0.815
54	0.716	0.839
55	0.754	0.864
56	0.796	0.889
57	0.841	0.916
58	0.890	0.943
59	0.943	0.971

This summary shows the figures that apply if a member retires precisely on his or her birthday; Appendix B contains the factors applying at any time between ages 50 and 60.

Voluntary early retirement without actuarial reduction

NHS employers may offer voluntary early retirement without any actuarial reduction of accrued benefits; however, they have to fund the extra costs incurred by waiving this reduction. (These costs cannot be met by the NHS pension scheme.) The employer must meet the cost of the pension from the date of retirement up to the normal retirement age of 60, as well as the cost of paying the lump sum before normal retirement age.

This option is not available to GPs as they do not have an employer.

However, the General Medical Services Committee of the BMA has asked the Health Department to consider ways in which this option could be made available to GPs.

Effect on other early retirement options

The new voluntary early retirement arrangements do not involve any enhancement of benefits, such as those available under ill-health retirement, redundancy, organizational change, retirement in the interests of the service and the 'achieving a balance' arrangements (see Table 10.1). It is important that those members who may be eligible for benefits under the enhanced arrangements are not persuaded to retire under voluntary early retirement arrangements. The Health Department has issued a circular to all NHS employers explaining that the new arrangements are entirely voluntary and should not be regarded as a substitute for existing arrangements.

Returning to work

Members taking voluntary early retirement cannot rejoin the NHS pension scheme. Nevertheless, if they return to NHS work, their pensions will be subject to abatement up until the age of 60 (see Chapters 15 and 16 for details). The NHS income earned after returning to work can, however, be pensioned through a personal pension plan (see Chapter 6).

11

Mental health officer/special class status

Special class status • Mental health officer (MHO) status • Management and academic posts • NHS pension scheme contributions paid by MHOs • Withdrawing MHO/special class status • Voluntary early retirement for MHOs/special class status members • Calculating MHO benefits

Special class status

Special class status originally applied to female NHS staff (extended to male staff from 17 May 1990) who are nurses, physiotherapists, midwives, health visitors or occupational health nurses. 'Nurse' in this context does not simply mean possessing a nursing qualification: it is essential that the work actually undertaken can be classified as nursing. Senior nurses with special class status may be able to retain this status if they move to a managerial/administrative post, providing a nursing qualification is an essential requirement of the new post. Members with special class status do not have to wait until the normal retirement age of 60 but may retire with full accrued benefits (and no actuarial reduction) from the age of 55 if they have held this status for at least the last five years of service. If male staff retire at the age of 55, the pension will be based on service since 17 May 1990 only; earlier service will be preserved for payment at age 60.

Mental health officer (MHO) status

MHOs are whole-time staff who devote the whole (or substantially the whole) of their time to the treatment of or caring for persons suffering from mental disorders. There are two key qualifying conditions, which must be satisfied in order to acquire this status.

- The person must be whole time; part-timers cannot be granted MHO status unless they are maximum part time. Two or more part-time posts taken together qualify for MHO status if they are whole time in total. MHO status is lost if the person switches from a whole-time to a part-time post, although MHO years accrued to date are retained for the purposes of entitlement to doubled years of service (see below).

- The 'whole or substantially the whole' of the person's time must be devoted to the care or treatment of mentally ill people.

This special status is intended to recognize the stress and strain of constantly caring for mentally ill patients. If there is any doubt, the NHS pensions agency has discretion to decide whether MHO status is appropriate.

MHOs with at least 20 years' MHO service have each year after 20 years counted double for pension purposes and may retire at age 55 onwards. Because the years of service are doubled, 40 years' service can be achieved by the age of 55, and 45 years by 58. Only *complete* years are doubled.

Service outside the NHS in MHO-type posts can be counted towards the 20 years' MHO service required to trigger the doubling. However, in these circumstances, doubling cannot begin until the age of 50 (whereas it can start immediately if over 20 years has been worked in the NHS itself). Any non-NHS service is, of course, not taken into account for pension purposes; its sole benefit is to count towards the achievement of 20 years' MHO service and thereby to allow doubling from age 50.

Box 11.1   Not such good advice

A psychiatrist with lengthy service asked his finance officer if it would make much difference to his pension if he dropped one session – from maximum part-time (10 sessions) to nine sessions. The answer was that he would only lose in pension $\frac{1}{11}$th of $\frac{1}{80}$th of salary for each year thereafter.

Perfectly good advice in most cases. Unfortunately, in this case it meant that the doctor lost mental health officer status and, with it, the opportunity to double all future years of service and to retire any time after the age of 55.

From the BMA's files

Management and academic posts

If staff give up some clinical work (ie the direct care of mentally ill people) to take on a managerial-type post, there is a danger that MHO status can be lost. This is because MHO status is intended to apply only if the person is continually caring for the mentally ill. However, discretion can be exercised; for example, if doctors give up no more than two clinical sessions, they can normally retain MHO status (provided they remain whole time or maximum part time within mental health). Likewise, an MHO taking up a post as a lecturer may be able to retain MHO status if the clinical sessions criterion is satisfied.

It is essential that anyone considering such posts should ascertain whether or not it will be possible to be credited with MHO status in the post. The NHS pensions agency has the final responsibility for deciding whether or not MHO status applies to the post.

Box 11.2   MHO status is not automatic

Dr K was denied mental health officer status on the grounds that during the period concerned, although he was full time, he only spent 70% of that time treating mentally ill people. This was technically true, in that 10% of his time was spent on training activities and 20% on research.

Closer examination showed, however, that the research consisted largely of the assessment of patients in terms of different possible forms of treatment and a follow-up of their subsequent progress. In other words, there was direct patient contact of a typically stressful MHO kind. The training activities were also in the mental health field.

The Pensions Agency was eventually persuaded that this doctor could not reasonably be assessed as anything other than 'spending the whole or substantially the whole of his time caring for mentally ill people', and MHO status was granted.

From the BMA's files

NHS pension scheme contributions paid by MHOs

Special contribution arrangements apply because the 'doubling factor' enables MHOs to reach maximum service earlier than other NHS staff:

• contributions must be paid until the age of 60 if service continues until then, even though the maximum service limit of 45 years may already have been reached

- contributions must cease at the age of 65
- contributions must cease on completion of 45 years' service if this occurs between the ages of 60 and 65.

MHOs may buy sufficient added years to take their actual and potential service, including doubling, to 40 years at the age of 55. These added years cannot themselves be doubled: they count as single years.

Withdrawing MHO/special class status

As part of the major review of the NHS pension scheme (see Chapter 16), from 6 March 1995 MHO/special class status is no longer available to new entrants to the scheme. The Health Department considered for some time that these special arrangements were no longer justified. Its decision to review the position was given impetus by a 1990 European Court judgement, which required that, in future, pension benefits should be accrued on an equal basis between the sexes, as a consequence of which, the special class concession (previously available only to female staff) had to be extended to male staff working in the same employment categories.

As far as MHO status was concerned, the Health Department's view was that it was an outdated concept (first introduced as part of the 1909 Asylum Act). The original purpose of these special early retirement arrangements was to ensure that eligible employees could retire at the age of 55 because of the highly demanding nature of their work. However, in practice, most of these staff retired much later than 55, their average retirement age being close to the normal retirement age of 60.

In withdrawing MHO/special class status for new entrants, the Health Department agreed that anyone holding this status on 6 March 1995 could retain it. If they lose it temporarily (eg because of a change of duties), they can reclaim it by returning to an eligible post, providing they have remained in the NHS pension scheme. Even if they leave the scheme, they can reclaim MHO/special class status if they return to the scheme within five years. Those who lost the status before 6 March 1995 will also be able to regain it if they stay in the NHS scheme or if they return to the scheme within five years of leaving it.

Voluntary early retirement for MHOs/special class status members

As far as retirement before age 55 is concerned, scheme members who retain MHO/special class status may apply for voluntary early retirement in the same way as other scheme members (see Chapter 10), but this is a most unattractive option because the Health Department insists that their pensions will be subject to the same actuarial reduction.

For example, an MHO on course to receive a full pension at the age of 55 only receives 0.716% of accrued pension if he or she retires at 54. The Health Department's view is that by retiring before 55, MHO status effectively no longer applies; thus the right to retire at 55 disappears and the normal actuarial reduction factor must apply as if 60 were the normal retirement age. In other words, MHOs retiring at the age of 54 will be treated as retiring six years early rather than only one year early.

Calculating MHO benefits

If an MHO continues working beyond the limit of 45 years' service, final benefits are calculated according to which of these two options is more favourable:

- pensionable salary calculated to the date 45 years' contributory service was completed, combined with all service up to that point, including doubled years. The resultant pension and lump sum are then increased by a factor to reflect inflation between the 45 years' service date and the last day of service

- pensionable salary calculated to the date of leaving service, based on all service up to that point but with no doubling of years.

12

Leaving or joining the NHS pension scheme: transfers and other options

> Leaving the NHS pension scheme • Transfers into the NHS pension scheme • To transfer or not to transfer?

Leaving the NHS pension scheme

A scheme member can leave by either leaving the NHS or remaining in the NHS but opting out of the scheme. On leaving, these options may be available:

- a refund of contributions
- preserving accrued benefits
- transferring accrued benefits to:
  - another occupational pension scheme
  - a personal pension plan (PPP)
  - an annuity contract (a buy-out bond).

Refund of contributions

A refund, which is only available to scheme members with less than two years' membership, should be avoided if possible (see Chapter 5). Members with less than two years' service can transfer benefits out of the scheme, although this option has to be carefully assessed.

Prior to 1988, when the 'two year' rule was introduced, it was possible for a refund to occur if someone left the NHS with more than two years' service, and many people lost considerable amounts of service as a result. In certain circumstances, it is possible to buy back this lost service at half price (see Chapter 5).

Preserving benefits

Members with more than two years in the scheme can leave their accrued pension and lump sum benefits in the scheme. No action is required because benefits are automatically preserved until age 60 unless a member requests otherwise. If the member becomes too ill to work, an ill-health pension is payable before the age of 60 (see Chapter 8).

If benefits are left in the scheme, they will be inflation proofed and increased each year in line with the retail prices index, which often makes this option attractive. Members may not do as well if they transfer benefits out of the scheme (see below).

Anyone likely to rejoin the scheme at some future date should note that their accrued service within the scheme will be preserved and automatically linked to any future NHS service. This means that, for GPs, superannuable income accrued up to the date of leaving the scheme will be dynamized in line with Review Body awards (see Chapter 3) during its years of preservation and added to the additional superannuable income earned after rejoining. For other scheme members, the earlier and later linked periods of service will all be pensioned at the salary rates prevailing at retirement age.

Transferring benefits

Anyone who transfers pension benefits as a result of changing jobs is often disappointed to find that they are credited with fewer years of service in the new scheme than they had accrued in the old one. Transfer arrangements are a major source of dissatisfaction, as is evident from the complaints received by the Occupational Pensions Advisory Service and the Pensions Ombudsman.

Transfer values

The value of a transfer is based on a cash equivalent of the accrued pension benefits. The transferee receives benefits based on an actuarial assessment of what that transfer value will buy in the receiving scheme. The NHS pension scheme bases all transfers on cash equivalence tables computed by the Government Actuary's Department. However, for various actuarial reasons, the NHS transfer value often does not buy the same number of years service in the receiving scheme. This problem is a common feature of transfers and is not unique to NHS cash equivalence tables.

Public sector transfer club

A loss of accrued service on transfer is less likely to arise (or its effect is lessened) if the transfer is between pension schemes that are members of the 'public sector transfer club'. The 'Club', as it is usually known, is a network of occupational pension schemes (largely in the public sector) that have collectively agreed to adopt a common approach to transfer values, thereby effectively eliminating certain unfavourable actuarial factors.

The NHS pension scheme is the largest scheme in the Club; other member schemes include:

- the Universities Superannuation Scheme

- the principal Civil Service pension scheme

- the armed forces pension scheme

- the Medical Research Council pension scheme.

Prior to 6 April 1988, a transfer between Club schemes normally guaranteed no loss on transfer; year-for-year service credit was usually given. However, since 1988, cash equivalence tables have been used to calculate transfer values, and it is now possible to lose service credit on transfer. Nevertheless, the benefits credited in the receiving scheme are usually very similar if it is a member of the Club.

Transfers out of the NHS pension scheme

NHS pension benefits can be transferred to:

- another occupational pension scheme

- a PPP

- an annuity contract (a buy-out bond).

Any recommendation to leave the NHS pension scheme and transfer benefits to a PPP should be treated with very great caution (see Chapter 5).

Members with two or more years in the scheme who are leaving NHS employment

A scheme member can transfer to another occupational pension scheme at any time before the age of 60. In order to transfer to a PPP or an annuity contract, the scheme member must have left the NHS and applied for the transfer by the age of 59, or within six months of leaving the pension scheme, whichever is later.

Members with less than two years in the scheme who are leaving NHS employment
Anyone transferring to an occupational pension scheme must join the new scheme within 12 months of leaving the NHS pension scheme and apply for a transfer within 12 months of joining the new scheme (or before the age of 60, whichever is sooner).

Anyone transferring to a PPP must do so before the age of 59, or within 12 months of leaving the NHS pension scheme, and apply for a transfer within 12 months of taking out the PPP.

Those transferring to an annuity contract can apply for a transfer at any time before the age of 59, providing they apply within 12 months of leaving the NHS.

Transferring NHS pension rights while remaining in NHS employment
This is not a wise thing to do in most cases (see Chapter 5), but a transfer to the types of pension arrangement outlined above is possible. However, if a member has two or more years NHS pension scheme membership before 6 April 1988, this pre-1988 service must be preserved in the NHS scheme until NHS employment ends. Any transfer will therefore be based on benefits earned since 6 April 1988 only.

Transfers into the NHS pension scheme

NHS staff must apply for the transfer in before the age of 60 and within 12 months of joining the scheme. It is possible to transfer in benefits from another occupational pension scheme or from a PPP.

Transfers within the NHS pension scheme, between England and Wales, Scotland and Northern Ireland

These transfers will be on a year-for-year credit basis. However, they must be applied for, in order to ensure that they actually take place and that the service record held by the appropriate pensions agency (see Appendix A) shows all NHS service.

To transfer or not to transfer?

The first step is to get a transfer value from the old scheme and to ask the receiving scheme what benefits this will buy. These benefits can be compared to the value of simply leaving a preserved benefit in the old scheme. This comparison is often difficult, particularly if the contemplated transfer is to a PPP whose future gains cannot be predicted and where comparing like with like is virtually impossible.

Several factors need to be taken into account when deciding whether to transfer.

- Is the scheme Club or non-Club (Club transfer is likely to be more favourable)?

- Future career plans (if you are likely to return to the NHS later, a transfer out may be ill advised).

- Are the receiving scheme's benefits index linked (most are in the public sector)? It is advisable to exercise considerable caution before transferring out benefits to a scheme whose benefits are not index linked.

- Age – a younger person can expect career and salary progression, including salary rises in excess of inflation, from the new employer; this would result in an attractive final pensionable salary, making a transfer the more favourable option. However, anyone approaching retirement is normally best advised to retain the security of index-linked preserved benefits.

If one is still in doubt after considering these and any other relevant factors, it may be wise to seek independent financial advice. Doctors who are BMA members can obtain independent financial advice from BMA Services Ltd (see Appendix A).

Transfers between the NHS pension scheme and the Universities Superannuation Scheme (USS)

The schemes have different normal retirement ages: 60 in the NHS and 65 in the USS. Thus a year's service in the NHS scheme is worth rather more than a year in the USS, because a full pension becomes available earlier in the former scheme. This means that a transfer from the USS to the NHS scheme will lead to a 'loss' of service credit, and a transfer in the other direction will lead to a 'gain'. However, the impact is reduced by the fact that, for transfer purposes, the USS uses a notional retirement age of 62.

Box 12.1   Loss on transfer – or was it?

Dr J, a male doctor, transferred from the NHS Scheme to the Universities Superannuation Scheme (USS) and back again. In doing so, he was upset to discover that he had 'lost' over a year of service. This seemed particularly odd because he understood that the first period of NHS service should have been transferred back into the NHS without loss and that the period of USS service should not have lost much value in transferring to the NHS.

A detailed examination of the figures showed that the problem was in fact the first period of NHS service, which lost value in transferring to the USS. Or did it? It was certainly worth less in years of service, but closer study showed that it was worth the same in terms of real value.

The service involved was pre-1972, and therefore the lump sum accruing from it at retirement would have been one times the pension, not three times (see Chapter 2 for details). However, the USS credited the doctor with a lump sum of three times pension. In order to pay for this, the service credit had to be reduced. On transferring back to the NHS, the service still attracted a lump sum at three times pension and therefore still needed to be based on reduced service.

The doctor had actually lost nothing.

From the BMA's files

Overseas transfers

It may be possible to transfer benefits into or out of the NHS pension scheme from or to an overseas scheme. Guidance should be sought from the NHS pensions agency and from the overseas scheme concerned.

Earnings cap

On transferring to a new scheme, members will be subject to the earnings cap; they cannot be pensioned on benefits in their new scheme above the earnings cap salary limit – £78 600 from April 1995 (see Chapter 1).

13

Three views on investing the NHS pension scheme lump sum

Investing your lump sum • The pitfalls of investing your lump sum

---

Investing your lump sum
John Winn

First comes the good news – the lump sum you receive from the NHS pension scheme is tax free. However, the bad news is not far behind, in that the tax man will try to get his share of any income or growth that the lump sum generates. Good investment advice will revolve around using simple, sensible and legal methods of keeping the tax man at bay.

To begin with, you should heed two excellent sayings:

- if something seems too good to be true, it probably is
- don't put all your eggs in one basket.

There are hundreds of schemes available, but before looking at the broad principles of these, you should consider some 'good housekeeping' tips. Your income in retirement is likely to be much lower than your pre-retirement salary. It is therefore important to plan.

First, look at all your assets and liabilities in order that the post-retirement planning can begin. Assets can be broken down into three broad categories:

- income
- fixed capital, eg property
- liquid capital.

This exercise provides the framework within which decisions for the short, medium and long term can be made.

Income

It is almost certain that you will not know what level of income you need until you have been retired for 12 or 18 months. It is, therefore, important to identify the main income sources and retain flexibility in your investments to cope with a changing income need.

The main sources of income are likely to be your NHS pension, your State pension, any personal pension plan (PPP) benefits and any work that you may do after retirement.

The NHS pension is important because it is protected against the ravages of inflation and, hopefully, you will have maximized your benefits from the scheme. If you have paid additional voluntary contributions (AVCs), either under the NHS or as a free-standing plan, the pension will have to be taken at the same time as your main NHS benefits. However, this income will either remain level throughout life or rise at a fixed rate, usually 3 or 5% per annum. Index-linked benefits are often too expensive to purchase in the private sector.

State pension benefits at present become payable from the age of 60 for women and 65 for men and, depending upon the type of benefit, have a large measure of inflation protection.

People who have utilized PPPs, or the old-style retirement annuities, will be faced with a range of options. First, should you take the benefits now or let them continue to roll up? If you are proposing to continue working, your income may support additional contributions towards such plans. Not only does this bring welcome tax relief on those contributions, but also the plans build up in a tax-free fund. So, if extra income is not needed immediately, this can be deferred until such time as you wish to give your finances an extra boost.

Second, when you do take the benefits, you will have the option to take some tax-free cash. This is usually a valuable option as the cash can be invested for future needs if income is not required immediately. Alternatively, if income is needed, the cash can be reinvested into income-generating vehicles, which are often more tax efficient than the pension plan.

Third, you should look at who can provide the best pension for the fund available under these plans. You do not have to take the pension offered by the investment house or insurance company who has run your plan. If an alternative, approved provider can give a higher benefit, you can elect to take the 'open market option' to this other company.

Finally, you will have a choice as to the type of pension you want. Is it to be level for life or should it escalate on a regular basis? Do you want some benefit to continue to be paid to your spouse in the event of your death?

If you are going to continue to do some work after retirement, how much income will this generate and for how long? Will this income be a salary from an employer such as the NHS or will it be 'private'? If it is private, remember that you may have to account for national insurance contributions and any tax due.

You should also take into account any income that is generated by your spouse. Is he or she at work and if so, how long will the employment last? If he or she is to retire or has already retired, is there an entitlement to any pension, State or private, in his or her own right?

Whilst income can be boosted by effective use of liquid capital, establishing regular income is important. Much of the income detailed above will be for life and some may be index linked. These are important benefits and provide a firm foundation for planning a capital investment programme.

By establishing who receives the income, yourself or your spouse, you also lay the foundation for making the most of separate taxation. This can be a very important exercise, as income tax rates vary from zero, if this is within your personal allowance, to 40% for higher levels. Each individual has a personal allowance, and a married couple has an additional allowance that can be moved to the person who has the highest income. Once the income exceeds the allowance, the next £3200 is taxed at 20%, the next £21 100 at 25% and anything in excess of this at 40%, for the 1995/96 tax year.

Often, liquid capital is used to generate additional income. Where possible, this capital should be held in the name of the individual who pays the lowest rate of tax. In this way, income that in one pair of hands might suffer a 40% rate can often bear a 20% or 25% rate, showing an immediate increase in value.

Fixed capital

For long-term planning, you should be aware of the value of those assets that cannot easily be disposed of, for example property, for both residential and holiday purposes, home contents, cars and major leisure items, such as boats. This listing establishes the core value of your estate, important for considering the impact of inheritance tax, and also ensures that running costs are brought into income calculations.

For example, do you still have a mortgage on your house? If so, when is it due to finish, will it be repaid by endowment policy or have you been repaying the capital regularly? It is not automatically right to use liquid capital to repay a mortgage. If your post-retirement income is sufficient to maintain the monthly repayment structure, other considerations may prevail. How much is your mortgage costing after allowing for the appropriate tax relief? Will investing your capital generate more income, particularly if you use your partner's allowances to reduce any income tax burden?

Do you have other loans? If you do, the interest charges are likely to be quite high and you should consider termination if the terms are reasonable.

Remember to put money aside for the renewal of items such as the car, fridge and TV.

Liquid capital

The final list covers capital available both now and in the future that can be used to generate income, growth or both. The NHS lump sum falls into this category and, any PPPs, or retirement annuities, will have an option to take part of the benefits in the form of a tax-free cash sum. In most cases, this option should be exercised to the maximum.

Full details should be obtained of all deposit accounts, whether bank or building society. How much is in each account? What is the present interest rate? What notice period is required for access? Are the accounts in your name, the name of your spouse or joint names?

Other sources of capital should be examined in similar detail. Many people own shares, often as a result of privatization issues or an inheritance, but do not review these holdings on a regular basis. When were the shares acquired and at what price? Do they generate an income and if so, how much? Do they have potential for future growth?

Holdings in unit trusts, personal equity plans (PEPs) and investment trusts must be detailed to assess income and growth possibilities. As with holdings in individual shares, members must be aware of the risks associated with stock market investments as well as their longer-term potential. One area often overlooked is the use of the capital gains tax (CGT) allowance to generate tax-free profit or income. Each person can generate real gains of up to £6000 in 1995/96 tax year that are exempt from CGT. Real gains are those that apply after allowing for the effects of inflation during the period the investment has been held.

National Savings certificates are another source of capital and often represent good growth with no risk. However, issues that have matured only earn interest at 3% at present, and members should look to reinvest in vehicles that give a better return.

Finally, you will need to look at regular savings plans that mature at retirement and in the years that follow. Many of these will provide a source of tax-free capital and, for some plans, the ability to take a tax-free income. It is useful to list the maturity of these plans to give a guide to future capital receipts.

Now what?

Armed with all the information on your financial position you can begin to plan.

In very brief terms, you will need to look at three time-related periods. First, what needs do you have for the next three years? This encompasses any capital expenditure and additional income. Investments to meet these items must be very secure and capable of being realized quickly. To this end, deposit accounts and cash-backed vehicles, for example cash unit trusts or sterling deposit accounts, are the most flexible. If your spouse has little or no income, much of the capital should be placed in their name to fully use their personal tax allowance. The 1995/96 allowance is £3525, and a 40% tax payer would need to generate a gross income of over £5800 to be left in the same net position. It is also important to remember that, providing you have your medium- and long-term investments properly organized, any extra income that you need in this period can be drawn from the capital in these accounts.

The second investment period will cover the four- to six-year timescale. In this area the use of guaranteed vehicles, such as National Savings certificates, will begin to replace the capital used in the early years. Other tax efficient plans, such as TESSAs, must also be considered. However, a small element of capital can also begin to be committed to non-deposit vehicles, where there is a greater element of risk but potential capital growth. Vehicles such as investment bonds or the new-style Capital Guarantee Bonds can be considered.

Finally, for periods in excess of six years, you may consider the more adventurous world of full equity investments. Here, unless you are able to commit large sums, you will spread the risk by using 'pooled' vehicles, such as unit trusts, and take advantage of any tax benefits, such as those available in PEPs.

The amount allocated to each of these time periods depends upon your needs and your willingness to accept a degree of risk with part of your capital. If you are averse to any form of risk, steer clear of stockmarket-related products, but remember that inflation eats away at your capital and you may be as well to take a small element of risk to overcome this.

Lastly, when you have set up your initial retirement plan, review the position regularly. This will enable you to take account of your changing circumstances, and your investment portfolio can be suitably adjusted.

Perhaps the best advice is to seek help from an independent financial adviser. They are required, by law, to act in your best interests and will guide you through the maze of investments, both throughout your working life and when you retire.

Investing your lump sum
Mike Rutherford

How would you invest £50 000? The answer to this seemingly simple question can, unfortunately, propel you into the highly complex, confusing world of financial advice. This comes with an apparently infinite number of answers and a dictionary full of the unintelligible jargon you would normally associate with trying to buy a computer or sending a rocket to Mars. Bid to offer, offer to bid, unit linked, PEP, unit trust, top slicing – what does it all mean and why is it made to sound so complicated?

Most people do not take note of the investment climate, or indeed where to go for financial advice, until some event in their life triggers the need. When I went to see a client recently retired, she was armed with building society leaflets, a National Savings booklet and details of the clearing bank Prime Gold Deposit rates. Mrs Jones had, not surprisingly, become progressively more confused as she juggled the various options and possibilities. To start to clear away from the confusion, we first had to establish three things:

1   her total financial circumstances including current capital, income and financial commitments

2   what, in principle, the money was to do; most people want capital growth, income, or a combination of the two

3   the types of investment that meet an acceptable risk profile. The major points to look for with all investments are accessibility, safety, tax efficiency, income potential, growth potential, investment choice and flexibility.

When considering what the money is to do, Mrs Jones has first to look at 'money timescale'. This means how much of the capital is wanted for instant access in the event of an emergency, how much is for the medium term, say 5–10 years, and how much is for the long term, 10 years plus. At her stage of life, she did not want to tie up the money over the long term. We then discussed the cash to be available for rapid access, the short-term money, and agreed that £10 000 should be put aside. We put £4000 of this into an instant access account with a high street building society and the £6000 balance into a building society postal account that paid a higher rate of interest.

We then talked about PEPs as the first part of a medium-term portfolio. Although surprised to learn that they fell into the medium- to high-risk profile, she felt that they were worth the risk because of the tax-free nature of the growth of the fund and because the proceeds were totally tax free. The maximum that can be put into a PEP in any tax year is £6000, so we decided that this would be a good route to take.

Having put some money in a reasonably speculative area, we now wanted to underpin the portfolio with some solid guarantees. We looked at a range of different options, starting with a with-profits bond. This product offers a yearly bonus on the capital that, once allocated, cannot be taken away (although some companies can invoke a market value adjuster if the capital is withdrawn within, for example, five years). As Mrs Jones is a basic rate taxpayer, it is highly unlikely that she would have to pay any tax on these proceeds. We also looked at National Savings income and option bonds, but as the interest on these products was taxable, it was decided to rule these out.

We then looked at a range of products that guarantee that the original capital investment cannot reduce in value, providing it is left invested for five years. The investment does, however, benefit from stock market growth. These products can vary tremendously and can cap the growth potential. This is primarily because the guarantees are expensive for the investment company to buy and their profit comes out of a share in the potential growth. From time to time, new products come onto the market, for a limited period or until the fund is fully subscribed. Guaranteed growth bonds have provided a range of guaranteed returns, regardless of movement in the FT–SE 100 index. The latest examples offer up to 11.5% of the original investment.

Mrs Jones felt that this approach was ideal for a portion of this money. It provided the necessary security with the potential for growth through an equity investment, and the proceeds would almost certainly be tax free, so £20 000 was allocated to this area.

Mrs Jones felt that as her superannuation income would meet all her day-to-day requirements, she would not necessarily need income from the capital. However, she wanted to have the flexibility, should this position change, that would enable her to create additional funds. Distribution bonds tend to be risk-averse funds, holding mainly fixed-interest securities, such as gilts, property and high yield UK equities. They provide an income that is derived from dividends paid on the stock held and not by cancellation of units in the fund. In simple terms, if you own a share, every year you get an income paid as a dividend, and if you need more income, you have to sell your share, ie cancel your unit.

However, even though you take the dividend, this does not stop the value of the share increasing. So with the distribution fund, the income does not prevent potential for capital growth, although not taking the income will increase the chances of capital growth. Whilst it carried no guarantees, the asset allocation or the areas into which the fund was invested were relatively safe and offered reasonable potential for growth. We allocated £10 000 into this area and elected not to take the income. Mrs Jones would review her pension and look at additional income in 6–12 months' time.

Providing Mrs Jones remains a basic rate tax payer, the proceeds of this fund will also be tax free. The maximum tax liability on the proceeds could only be at the difference between the higher rate (40%) and basic rate tax (25%), namely 15%.

We had by now allocated £46 000 of the original £50 000. With the remaining £4000, Mrs Jones would take a more speculative or high-risk approach. We examined a wide rage of unit trusts, which incorporated small UK companies, Japan, the Asian basin, the Pacific basin, technology funds, Australia and Latin America. Rather than invest in any one of these areas, thus putting 'all the eggs in one basket', it was felt best to invest in an emerging markets fund, which spread the investment over a range of these and similar funds. Unit trusts, unlike the other areas we looked at, have a potential CGT liability. The annual allowance, currently £5800, before it becomes payable means that, with careful management, Mrs Jones is unlikely to have to pay CGT on the investment. It is worth mentioning that the allowance of £5800 does not roll over from year to year. If it is not used in any one tax year, it is lost.

In summary, Mrs Jones invested £50 000 to meet a wide range of needs. As a contingency fund (short term), she allocated £10 000: £6000 into a building society postal account and £4000 into an instant access building society account. A PEP took up £6000, and £30 000 was put into medium-term investment: £20 000 with growth guarantees and £10 000 into risk-averse distribution bonds. Finally, £4000 was invested into the emerging markets fund.

This case study represents a typical client's needs, but, of course, every individual has a unique set of circumstances and the personal situation must be examined in detail. In this area, usually of long-term financial planning, mistakes can be costly, and the need for professional, independent and impartial financial advice is highly recommended.

The pitfalls of investing your lump sum
Peter Scott-Malden CB

So, retirement is only a few months away, and you are already starting to dream about that munificent lump sum and what you are going to do with it. Well, the first thing to do is to make sure you actually get it, on the day when its due – even the best administrative machines have been known to make a muddle. You are the one who will suffer, so check up that the wheels are turning as they should.

When the great day does come, unless you are a very well-organized person, put the money away in a building society or a deposit account until you are ready to make your long-term investment decisions. You will almost certainly be wise to consult a financial adviser, preferably one who is independent and who can survey the whole market. But before you do that, do some serious thinking about your investment objectives. Will you have to rely on income from your investments? Or do you primarily need capital growth? How much risk are you prepared to accept? Are you going to need rapid access to your money? Are you prepared to lock up your money for years or do you wish to retain some flexibility? These are the sorts of question that any adviser worth his salt will ask before he can start to give you advice.

Inflation may not look too serious at present (1995), but historically, since at least 1945, it has been wise, when making long-term investment plans, to assume average annual inflation of the order of 5%. This rate has the effect of *halving*, in 13 years, the purchasing power of money deposited with, for instance, a building society, or indeed in most National Savings products. Thirteen years may seem a long time, but people retiring this year have substantial life expectations (Table 13.1).

Table 13.1 Life expectancies at retirement

Age at retirement	Life expectancy (years)	
	Female	Male
60	23	$18\frac{1}{2}$
65	19	15
70	15	12

One line of defence against inflation is the National Savings index-linked savings certificate; the current 7th Issue gives complete protection (after the first year) against any rise in the retail prices index since the purchase date, and also a bonus of 3% compound if held for the full five years (less if cashed in earlier). However, most people seeking protection from inflation will be looking to invest at least a part of their lump sum in companies that, by component management and expansion, can hope to achieve genuine increases in the value of their assets and thus in their share prices.

Direct investment in the stock market is for those who already know their way around or who have sufficient money to make it worth while buying regular professional supervision. The majority will prefer indirect investment by means that will lessen their risk but still give them some prospect of capital growth – normally unit trusts, investment bonds or investment trusts. Although technically very different from each other, all of these operate by pooling money from large numbers of investors and then investing it in a spread of underlying securities, usually the ordinary shares of perhaps 50 or 100 companies in the UK or overseas.

Unit trusts are straightforward. You buy at one price and sell at another, about 5–6% less, both readily ascertainable in the press. Dividends are subject to income tax and paid with tax deducted. Gains are subject to CGT, but this is unlikely to be a serious factor while the annual personal CGT allowance is over £5000. The management company is not subject to any tax on its own operations.

Investment bonds take the form of a single premium life assurance policy, which can be written on the joint lives of a couple. The buying and selling process is similar to that of unit trusts, except that more information is required on the proposal form. Income is normally reinvested, but the investor can draw up to 5% of his original investment as income for 20 years with no immediate deduction of tax; basic rate tax is, in any case, borne by the insurance company, and any realized capital gain, or income drawn above the 5% level, is subject only to the margin of higher rate income tax (currently 15%), and then only if the investor is liable after a complex process known as 'top slicing'.

Investment bonds differ from unit trusts in being subject to CGT on their own operations and will therefore normally produce an inferior performance on similar underlying investments. Accordingly, for most investors, unit trusts are preferable, except for someone to whom the special features of investment bonds are important – notably the ability to defer higher rate tax on 5% annual income and the freedom offered by most bonds to switch very cheaply between the different funds held under the bond's 'umbrella'.

Investment trust companies (properly so called) do a similar job but in a significantly different way. They are companies whose business is to invest in other companies, and the investor actually buys shares in the investing company. Consequently, the value of the investment will vary not only with the performance of the underlying investments (as in the case of unit trusts and investment bonds), but also with the standing of the company itself in the stock market. The standing of the company may be further affected – for good or ill – by the company's use of borrowed money in addition to shareholder's funds. Investment trusts offer many special features, such as split-level trusts, zero-dividend preference shares and savings schemes, but it must be realized that they are not directly comparable to unit trusts and that investors are dipping at least a toe directly in the waters of the stock market.

PEPs deserve a word. Their advantage is that investments are free of both income tax and CGT; on the other hand, you have to pay your plan manager, and his charges roughly offset the income tax savings, at least for basic rate tax payers. Moreover you cannot go liquid – you must remain fully invested in the UK stock market or you lose the tax advantages. If a plan is held for a number of years, the CGT exemption will become more important. Moreover if your chosen unit or investment trust can be held in a PEP without additional charge – as many can – or even with a discount, it is clearly sensible to take advantage of the tax savings. However, beware of letting the tax tail wag the investment dog.

One other tax angle should be mentioned – the independent taxation of spouses. If the spouse has a lower or negligible income, there may be substantial tax savings to be achieved by arranging that the investment income accrues to the spouse, in order to take advantage of the spouse's personal allowance and/or basic rate tax band. (Spouses also have a separate CGT allowance.) However, be careful – both the capital and the income must be fully and legally under the spouse's own control.

Annuities are sometimes recommended, but are seldom good value (especially at present interest rates) until you are well into your seventies or even eighties. Above all, they are the most inflexible investment there is.

The best way of choosing a financial adviser is by recommendation. However, you may still be faced with the question of how he or she should be remunerated. Most still work on a commission basis, but this inevitably introduces the possibility of bias (for example, insurance companies normally pay better commission than unit trust management companies); however, more and more are now offering a fee basis. This may seem more expensive – although any commission received ought to be rebated against the fee – but it does tend to establish a more lasting relationship, which may be to your long-term benefit.

Finally, security. Obviously, National Savings are satisfactory – or we are all in trouble! Your building society should be a participant in the compensation scheme of the Building Societies Association. Insurance companies should be individually checked, although there is a Policy Hold-ers' Protection Board, which guarantees 90% of your original investment. Unit trusts are closely supervised. Make sure that your financial adviser is duly authorized by the appropriate regulatory body and that clients' money is segregated in a separate account. If the worst comes to the worst, there is an Investors' Compensation Scheme set up by the Securities and Investments Board (see Appendix A), who will send you, on request, five interesting booklets on aspects of investor protection.

14

Other public sector pension schemes

The Universities Superannuation Scheme (USS) • The
Principal Civil Service Pension Scheme (PCSPS) • The
Armed Forces Pensions Scheme (AFPS) • The Medical
Research Council Pension Scheme (MRCPS)

The vast majority of people working in the medical field are in the NHS
pension scheme. However, a minority are members of other public
sector pension schemes. This chapter outlines the main features of some
of these other schemes. Further information is available from each
scheme's booklet or administrators, and from employers.

This chapter covers the following schemes:

- the Universities Superannuation Scheme
- the Civil Service pension scheme
- the armed forces pension scheme
- the Medical Research Council pension scheme.

and describes the following features:

- contributions
- pension
- lump sum
- retirement age
- dependants' benefits
- early retirement
- additional benefits
- indexation
- sources of further information.

The Universities Superannuation Scheme (USS)

Contributions

Employees pay 6.35% of salary (6.0% towards the main scheme and 0.35% for additional benefits on ill-health retirement and death in service). The employer contributes the balance of the cost of scheme benefits.

The scheme is funded; in other words, contributions are invested and the investment fund is used to pay benefits (unlike the NHS pension scheme which is notionally funded – see Chapter 1 for an explanation of 'notional' funding). Like all funded occupational pension schemes, trustees are appointed to oversee the administration of the scheme.

Pension

A pension of $\frac{1}{80}$th of pensionable salary is payable for each year of service, subject to a maximum of $\frac{40}{80}$ths at the age of 65.

Lump sum

The tax-free lump sum is three times the pension.

Retirement age

Normal retirement age is age 65.

Dependants' benefits

Death in service
If a scheme member dies, a pension is payable to the surviving spouse and qualifying children. If death occurs in service, the spouse's pension is 50% of the pension the member would have received at the age of 65 (plus a further 25% for each child, up to a maximum of two children). An enhanced lump sum is also payable.

Death after retirement
The same percentages are payable as for death in service, but the benefits are based on the member's actual pension at the date of death. In some circumstances, a lump sum may also be payable.

Early retirement

Ill health
Providing five years' scheme membership has been completed, an enhanced pension and lump sum are payable as if the member had worked to the age of 65 (maximum of 40 years' service). A basic, unenhanced pension is payable if service is between two and five years in length.

Redundancy
An enhanced pension and lump sum may be payable, if the employer is willing to fund the costs of the enhancement.

Voluntary early retirement
Normal retirement age is 65, but it may be possible to retire from the age of 60 if the employer agrees, or without the employer's agreement with an actuarially reduced pension.

Additional benefits

It is possible, within the usual limits (see Chapter 5), to pay additional contributions in order to buy added years of service or to pay into an additional voluntary contributions (AVC) contract or a free-standing voluntary contributions (FSAVC) contract.

Indexation

Pensions are increased each year in line with the increase in the retail prices index (early retirement pensions, other than ill-health pensions, not being indexed until the age of 55).

Sources of further information

The USS publishes 'A Guide for Members', which can be obtained from employers. The USS can be contacted directly at the address shown in Appendix A.

The Principal Civil Service Pension Scheme (PCSPS)

Contributions

Although the PCSPS is sometimes looked upon as a 'non-contributory' scheme, there is an employee contribution rate of 1.5%, mainly in respect of widow's/widower's benefits.

Pension

A pension of $\frac{1}{80}$th of pensionable salary is payable for each year of service, up to $\frac{40}{80}$ths at the age of 60 (normal retirement age) or $\frac{45}{80}$ths at 65 or over.

Lump sum

The tax-free lump sum is three times the pension. (This will be reduced if there are outstanding survivors' pension contributions – see below.)

Retirement age

Normal retirement age is 60, but it is possible to build up benefits after that age up to a total of 45 years' service.

Dependants' benefits

Widowers' benefits are based only on service since 1987, unless prior service was purchased. The position in respect of widows' benefits is more complicated and depends upon contributions paid prior to 1978 when full-rate contributions became compulsory. The following summary assumes full-rate widows' benefits and post-1987 widowers' benefits.

Death in service
The spouse's pension is 50% of the enhanced pension that the member would have received if retired on the grounds of ill health on the date of death (see 'Ill-health retirement' below). Children's pensions are also payable in respect of qualifying children, at the rate of 25% for each child, up to a maximum of 50%. A lump sum of twice pensionable salary is also payable.

Death after retirement
The same percentages are payable as for death in service, but the benefits are based on the member's actual pension at the date of death. In some circumstances, a lump sum may also be payable.

Early retirement

Ill health
Providing service is more than five years, enhancement is similar to that in the NHS pension scheme (Table 14.1). The pension and lump sum are based on this enhanced service.

Table 14.1 PCSPS: ill-health retirement

Service	Service enhancement
Less than 10 years	Doubled (limit: age 65)
10 or more years	Increased to 20 years (limit: age 65) *or,* if better, $6\frac{2}{3}$ years (limit: age 60)

Compulsory early retirement (including redundancy)
For those aged 50 and over with more than five years' service, service is enhanced by $6\frac{2}{3}$ years and a pension and lump sum are payable. In addition, there is a lump sum compensation payment.

For those under the age of 50, with more than two years' service, a preserved pension and lump sum are payable at 60. In addition, a lump sum compensation payment is payable.

Flexible early retirement
This is a voluntary arrangement enabling management to invite individuals to retire early. For those aged 50 and over with more than five years' service, the benefits are the same as for compulsory early retirement (see above) but with no lump sum compensation payment. For those under the age of 50, with more than two years' service, a preserved pension and lump sum are payable at 60. In addition, a lump sum compensation payment is payable.

Approved early retirement
This enables departments with surplus staff to seek volunteers to retire early (subject to certain age and service limitations). The pension and lump sum are paid immediately and are based on accrued service only.

Actuarially reduced retirement

Employees aged 50 or over may opt to retire early with an actuarially reduced pension and lump sum. The actuarial reduction for each year that benefits are paid earlier than the due retirement age is approximately 5% for the pension and 2.5% for the lump sum.

Additional benefits

It is possible, within the usual limits, to buy added years or to pay into an AVC or FSAVC contract.

Indexation

Pensions are increased each year in line with the increase in the retail prices index (early retirements, other than for ill health, not being increased until the age of 55).

Sources of further information

The PCSPS publishes several useful leaflets on the scheme. The address and telephone number of the Civil Service Pensions Department is in Appendix A.

The Armed Forces Pensions Scheme (AFPS)

Contributions

Because the AFPS is a non-contributory scheme, there are no employee contributions. However, the Review Body on armed forces' pay takes account of the value of pension benefits when recommending pay rates.

Pensionable pay

Pension benefits in the AFPS are not based directly on an individual's pay but on representative rates of pay for each rank and length of service.

Pension

Officers with 16 years' service, and other ranks with 22 years' service, are entitled to an immediate pension on retirement at any age. For officers, the pension is 28.5% of representative pay after 16 years, rising uniformly to 48.5% after 34 years' service. For other ranks, it is 31.833% of representative pay after 22 years, rising to 48.5% after 37 years' service.

Lump sum

The tax-free lump sum is three times the pension.

Retirement age

There is no fixed retirement age. Benefits become payable after 16 or 22 years' service (see above). However, the normal retirement age is 55, in that maximum benefits can be achieved at that age.

Dependants' benefits

Death in service
Benefits are based on the pension the member would have received if retired on the grounds of ill health on the date of death (see below). This, in turn, depends on whether or not death was attributable to service. The spouse may receive 50% of the member's pension, with an additional 25% payable in respect of each qualifying child, up to a maximum of two children.

Death after retirement
The same percentages are paid as for death in service, but based on the member's pension at date of death.

Different arrangements may apply for service before 1 April 1973.

Early retirement

Ill health

- *Illness not attributable to service.* For those with five or more years' service, a pension and lump sum are payable based on rank, years of service and a percentage of full career pension.

- *Illness attributable to service.* In addition to the 'non-attributable' pension and lump sum, an extra pension and lump sum are payable based on rank and degree of disability, irrespective of length of service (and irrespective of AFPS membership).

Other reasons
Benefits are payable after 16 years' (officers) or 22 years' (other ranks) service.

Additional benefits

It is possible to pay extra contributions to purchase added years to achieve maximum service at the age of 55, or to pay into an AVC or FSAVC contract.

Indexation

Although the Pensions Increase Act (which enables most public sector schemes to increase pensions in line with inflation) does not apply to the AFPS, pensions are increased in the same way, ie they are increased each year in line with the retail prices index (but not until the age of 55, except for ill-health and dependants' pensions).

Sources of further information

The AFPS publishes two useful booklets (AFPS 1 and AFPS 2). Further information can be obtained directly from the relevant service department (see Appendix A).

The Medical Research Council Pension Scheme (MRCPS)

Contributions

Scientific staff pay 6.75% of salary (6.0% towards the main scheme and 0.75% towards a supplementary scheme, which funds enhanced ill-health retirement and death benefits). Other staff (except maintenance staff) contribute 6.5% (6.0% to the main scheme and 0.5% to the supplementary scheme). Maintenance staff contribute 5.5% (5.0% to the main scheme and 0.5% to the supplementary scheme). The MRC pays the balance of the cost of the scheme.

The scheme is funded; ie contributions are invested and the investment fund is used to pay benefits. Trustees oversee the operation of the scheme.

Pension

A pension of $\frac{1}{80}$th of pensionable salary is payable for each year of service, subject to a maximum of $\frac{40}{80}$ths at normal retirement age (see below) and $\frac{45}{80}$ths in total.

Lump sum

The tax-free lump sum is three times the pension.

Retirement age

Normal retirement age is 65 for scientific staff and 60 for other staff.

Dependants' benefits

Death in service
Spouses' and childrens' pensions are payable; the spouse receives 50% of the member's ill-health pension (see below) and children 25% each (up to a maximum of two children). An enhanced lump sum is also payable.

Death after retirement
The same percentages are payable as for death in service, but the benefits are based on the member's actual pension at date of death. In some circumstances, a lump sum may also be payable.

Early retirement

Ill-health retirement
Pension and lump sum benefits are based on service enhanced to normal retirement age.

Compulsory early retirement
For those aged 50 and over, with five or more years' service, service is enhanced by up to $6\frac{2}{3}$ years and a pension and lump sum are payable. In addition, there is a lump sum compensation payment.

For those under the age of 50, with more than two years' service, a preserved pension and lump sum are payable at normal retirement age (see above). In addition, a lump sum compensation payment is payable.

Flexible early retirement
This is a voluntary arrangement enabling management to invite individuals to retire early. For those over the age of 50, with five or more years' service, the benefits are the same as for compulsory early retirement, except that the additional lump sum compensation payment is not payable. For those under the age of 50, with two or more years' service, a preserved pension and lump sum are payable at normal retirement age. In addition, a lump sum compensation payment is payable.

Approved early retirement
This enables management to seek volunteers for early retirement, subject to certain age and service limitations. The pension and lump sum are payable immediately but are based on accrued service only.

Actuarially reduced early retirement
Employees aged 50 and over, with two or more years' service, may retire early with an actuarially reduced pension and lump sum. The actuarial reduction, for each year that benefits are paid early is approximately 5% for the pension and 2.5% for the lump sum.

Additional benefits

It is possible to pay extra contributions to purchase added years or to contribute to an AVC or FSAVC contract.

Indexation

Pensions are increased each year in line with the retail prices index (early retirement pensions, other than for ill health, not being indexed until the age of 55).

Sources of further information

The MRCPS publishes a members' booklet, which is available from employers. Further information can be obtained directly from the MRC (see Appendix A).

15

Working after retirement

Working in the NHS – Abatement • Working outside the NHS

For many, retiring is a difficult experience, not only because there is usually a reduction in income, but also because of other more subjective factors, which are often difficult to recognize and articulate. There is the sudden change from having very little leisure time to having almost too much free time. Perhaps, more importantly, there is a great sense of loss – both of status and purpose – when a lifelong career ends. These feelings can affect even those individuals who have planned for their retirement and have positively welcomed it. This experience can be described in various ways: a loss of a role, status, prestige, meaning to life; no longer being of service to others; no longer commanding the respect, even admiration, of one's peers and patients. It is not through a foolish arrogance or misplaced self-importance that many people sense these kinds of loss. A working life is a formidable commitment from which it is not always easy to walk away.

Individuals cope with this sense of loss in a number of ways, depending upon their temperament and personality. A helpful way of coping with the problem is purposefully to set about establishing a new role and new way of living in retirement. This may be as simple as developing one's favourite leisure activities (see Chapter 20). On the other hand, it can also sometimes be helpful to continue to work after retirement (albeit part time), so that the jump from full-time work to full-time leisure is not nearly as sudden and can be adjusted to gradually, from both a financial and a psychological viewpoint.

This chapter looks at some of those matters that need to be taken into account in returning to work after retirement.

Working in the NHS

It is possible to return to work in the NHS after retirement. However, it is necessary to consider carefully the question of abatement.

Abatement

An NHS pension is abated (ie reduced or taken away completely) if, on returning to work after retirement, the post-retirement income plus the pension exceeds the pre-retirement income.

Whom does abatement affect?
Major changes were made to the abatement rules with effect from 6 March 1995.

Abatement does not apply to anyone retiring after 6 March 1995 if:

- they take a significant break in employment before returning to work (at least one month). If they do not take a break of at least one month, the pension will be withdrawn completely for the period of re-employment (irrespective of the level of post-retirement income). It is not necessary to take a break from a continuing concurrent post of less than 16 hours per week

- they are aged 60 or over. Scheme members receiving a pension for any reason before the age of 60 will continue to be abated until 60.

Abatement will not apply to anyone who retired before 6 March 1995 but returned to work after that date, provided that there has been a break in employment of at least one month.

Members already being abated at 6 March 1995 will continue to be abated until they retire again, at which point the new rules will apply to them and they will not be abated in future, subject to the restrictions described above.

From 6 March 1995, it is not possible to rejoin the NHS pension scheme on being re-employed (the only exception being those scheme members who retire on health grounds and are re-employed before the age of 50). However, it will be possible to take out a personal pension in respect of the post-retirement income.

How does abatement work?
Even after 6 March 1995, a considerable number of scheme members will continue to be subject to abatement, including:

- anyone under the age of 60

- anyone already being abated at 6 March 1995 who has not subsequently retired again.

Figure 15.1 illustrates how abatement operates for these members.

'Pay' for this purpose means NHS superannuable income; non-NHS income is ignored, together with any NHS income that is not superannuable.

The lump sum is not abated. It is possible to gain access to the tax-free lump sum by retiring temporarily, even though the pension itself is abated or withdrawn.

Abatement continues until final retirement but not beyond the age of 70.

Abatement still applies if the member either opts out of the NHS pension scheme on re-employment or cannot pay any more contributions because maximum service has been achieved. It also applies to those members who are contributing to the scheme under the 'direction arrangements' (see Chapter 5), although, in their case, opting out of the scheme on re-employment enables them to avoid abatement.

Box 15.1   Opting out would have avoided abatement

Dr A was able to contribute to the NHS pension scheme under the 'direction' arrangements, even though his employer was non-NHS. He retired but decided to return to work. He wondered whether opting out of the NHS scheme at that point might be sufficient to avoid abatement. A mix-up ensued between the employer's pension officer and the pensions agency, with the result that Dr A was told that he would be abated whether or not he opted out. He therefore decided not to opt out and to rejoin the pension scheme.

Three years and £75 000 worth of lost pension later, Dr A discovered that this advice was wrong: opting out would have been sufficient to make sure that his pension was not abated.

After some little struggle, Dr A managed to have his position restored: his abated pension was returned to him, along with a refund of contributions for the three years he had rejoined the scheme.

From the BMA's files

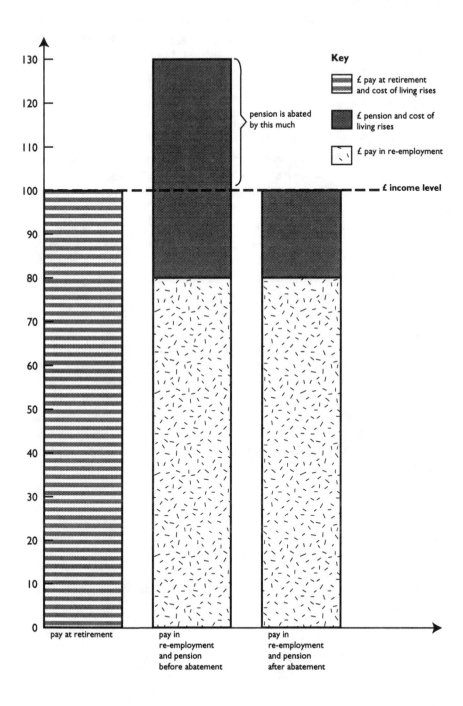

Figure 15.1   How abatement works

Earnings margin
This is the amount of income that can be earned on re-employment without the NHS pension being abated (at retirement, the Paymaster General's Office tells you how much this is). Look out for this important information because it helps you to assess possible NHS re-employment.

Method of assessment
In addition to the changes explained above, for those still subject to abatement, the rules were relaxed in a significant way with effect from 6 March 1995. In future, the abatement assessment will be calculated on an annual basis; thus, abatement will only occur if, throughout a full year, income plus pension taken together exceed the annual rate of pre-retirement income.

This is a valuable improvement to the scheme. Previously, the nature of the member's income on re-employment made a significant difference to the abatement position. Members on fixed incomes were abated whatever the length of their employment; ie if their new income plus pension over this period exceeded pre-retirement income, they were abated. Working occasionally as a locum, for instance, could have resulted in full abatement.

However, if the income earned after retirement was variable, the abatement was calculated on a quarterly basis, thus reducing the chances of short-term re-employments being abated. It was possible to introduce a 'variable' income in a number of ways, for example if a doctor was required to be available for domiciliary visits or to work on an 'as and when' basis. In these circumstances, it may well have been possible to work on full pay for, for example, six weeks in a particular quarter and to avoid being abated.

Pre-retirement income
The higher a member's pre-retirement income, the less likely he or she is to be abated on re-employment. Pre-retirement income is defined as whichever is the higher of:

- *either* actual income in the best of the last three years before retirement

  or

- actual income at the date of retirement (plus any superannuable fees paid during the previous 12 months).

Practitioners

For practitioners, the normal pre-retirement figure used for abatement purposes is the annual average of the total uprated (dynamized) superannuable income.

However, if a GP retires from a hospital post (eg a clinical assistant post) but continues as a GP, the pre-retirement earnings figure consists of the clinical assistant income plus the GP income, although the latter is calculated differently, in this case being the average of the last three years' dynamized income and not the average of the total dynamized income.

It may, of course, be possible to return to work on a reduced share of the profits in order to avoid or reduce abatement.

Box 15.2   Abatement harshly applied

Dr M was a GP. She developed health problems and reluctantly decided that she would need substantially to reduce her hours of work. She therefore left her practice and took a post as a part-time clinical assistant. Unfortunately, after several years, her health deteriorated further and she decided to take ill-health retirement.

Because her GP post had finished more than 12 months before she retired, her pre-retirement earnings for abatement purposes excluded the GP income (despite this being her main income as a doctor) and was based solely on her clinical assistant sessions. As a result, although her health permits her to do some occasional NHS locums, her pension would be fully abated whenever she did so.

Dr M should have applied for ill-health retirement when she first became ill; she is effectively being punished for her courage in struggling on in a lower-paid post.

From the BMA's files

Cost of living increases

The pre-retirement earnings figure is increased each year in line with the increase awarded to pensions, ie the retail prices index increase.

Increased benefits following re-employment

After 6 March 1995, it is not possible to rejoin the NHS pension scheme following retirement (except for those who have retired on health grounds and are re-employed before the age of 50). However, members who have rejoined in the past will have built up additional benefits. When they finally retire, their pensions will be calculated using whichever of these methods produces the better result:

- the existing pension is terminated and a new one is calculated using final pensionable salary plus all previous service (using, for GPs, total superannuable income dynamized up to the final retirement date).

  or

- a separate pension is calculated for the re-employed period of service and added to the earlier pension (increased since the first retirement in line with the cost of living).

If there is doubt as to which method produces the better result, the member is given the option of choosing between them.

After 6 March 1995, the first method above is only available to those members who were re-employed before that date and retired afterwards. If they come back to work again after their second retirement, they will be in the same position as other members; they cannot rejoin the scheme and they will not be abated, but the first method will not be available when they finally retire.

This first method will continue to be available to members with pre-served pensions, ie those who left the NHS but did not take a pension and still have accrued benefits in the scheme. When they return to the NHS, their new service will link up with the preserved service from their earlier employment.

Re-employment after receiving an enhanced pension

If members had received enhanced years of service on retirement (eg because of having retired on redundancy grounds, etc), the option of rejoining the scheme may not have been advisable. This is because the enhanced years of service will not be double counted. For example, if service was enhanced by five years, during the first five years of re-employment, there will be no extra service credit accruing. However, if members in this position did rejoin, it is likely that some extra pension would be payable because benefits would be recalculated on a higher final salary.

The position for those who retired on an enhanced ill-health pension is likely to be more favourable because it is possible to retain the ill-health pension and to receive an additional credit for the re-employed years.

Working outside the NHS

Paid work

Unemployment remains high, and the proportion of people over the age of 55 in full-time work has dropped significantly in recent years. Redundancy, either voluntary or compulsory, has had an effect on employment levels, and many people have taken advantage of good employer occupational pension schemes to leave work before the State pension age (60 for women and 65 for men). Therefore, full-time jobs are often hard to find, and retired people face an additional problem because many employers discriminate on grounds of age against older people.

However, there has been an increase in the number of casual and part-time jobs (albeit often at the lower paid end of the market), and some employers actively seek older workers because of their maturity, skills and experience, and the fact that they may not be subject to the protection of employment legislation.

Where to look

Many retired doctors already undertook private work while still working in the NHS; their post-retirement working may simply involve continuing with that work and allowing it to diminish steadily until they eventually decide to retire completely from medical practice.

For others, post-retirement work may require an active job search and even a complete change in the type of work undertaken. For example, a more modest job may be easier to find and sufficiently rewarding.

In the search for a post-retirement job, you are likely to need an up-to-date curriculum vitae (CV), which is presented in a way that takes account of the type of job you are looking for. You should also think about how to present yourself at interview, taking into account your previous experience and the type of job you are seeking. In short, strange as it may seem, the task of job-hunting for a mature and experienced person in their 50s and 60s involves the same basic discipline and tasks as it does for the school leaver or young graduate.

Possible ways of searching for a job include:

- *employment agencies*: these often specialize in particular types of employment, and although they cannot expect to place everyone, their income depends on finding work for people, by charging the prospective employer rather than the job-hunter. Telephone directories list those operating in the local area

- *job centres*: it may be worth making contact with your local job centre (which tends to be used by smaller and more local employers), not only for job vacancies, but also for details of the help that is available in searching for a job. If you are under 60, you may wish to 'sign on' in order to ensure that you are credited with national insurance contributions towards your State pension (see Chapter 17)

- *direct response to advertisements*: this can be a soul-destroying experience, particularly if you receive many refusals. Nevertheless, a well-prepared CV and brief, well-presented, covering letter can greatly increase your chances. You may wish to seek professional advice on how to present this material

- *writing to prospective employers*: this approach is feasible if you know of employers interested in people with your skills and/or who discriminate in favour of older people

- *personal contacts*: jobs can come from the most unexpected quarter, and it is sensible to let friends, relatives, colleagues and neighbours know that you are interested in working after retirement.

Voluntary work

A common feeling among people at the end of a career that has been personally, and even financially, rewarding is that they would like to 'put something back in'. In other words, they feel that society has, on the whole, been good to them and that they wish in return to make a contribution to the community, for which they require no reward other than personal satisfaction. This personal satisfaction can, of course, mean a great deal and can help to overcome the sense of loss that may occur when a career ends. Voluntary work can fill precisely this gap, offering a sense of purpose, appreciation from colleagues and clients and a new source of self-esteem and professional fulfilment. It can also provide an opportunity for one to contribute to a cause which one believes to be worth while.

The variety of organizations that are keen to receive voluntary help is truly extensive, and it is well beyond the scope of this book to attempt even to list them. Many people will have their own interests and priorities and will know exactly where to go. For those who are uncertain or who would like to explore the options in more detail, the following might be a good starting point.

- *Citizens Advice Bureaux.* In addition to using thousands of volunteers themselves, they are a good source of information about other groups wanting volunteers.

- *Local library.* This is a useful resource for retired people in a variety of ways and should be able to provide information about local groups wanting voluntary workers.

- REACH (retired executives action clearing house – see Appendix A). This finds part-time voluntary work for retired people with professional skills.

- *The local phone book.* A quick look under the heading 'Voluntary organizations' in the local telephone directory should yield a surprisingly long and varied list of groups in the area who are looking for voluntary help.

16

Changes to the NHS pension scheme

Major changes in the NHS pension scheme take effect from 6 March 1995 in England and Wales, and from 1 April 1995 in Scotland and Northern Ireland. These changes have been the subject of consultations between the Health departments and health service trade unions. The Departments also consulted the Treasury and other Civil Service departments. The Treasury insisted that the changes had to be 'cost neutral', and the scheme's actuaries (the Government Actuary's Department) have confirmed that the overall package satisfies this requirement.

In previous chapters, we have described how these changes affect particular aspects of the NHS pension scheme. However, because of their importance, this chapter provides a general summary and commentary on them.

1 The death in service lump sum increases to two times annual salary, and there are no deductions for pre-1972 service.

This brings the NHS scheme in line with the best public sector schemes (although it remains behind the private sector, where the lump sum is usually at least $2\frac{1}{2}$ or three times annual salary). Nevertheless, it is a real and significant improvement to the scheme's 'insurance-type' benefits.

The maximum lump sum payable was previously $1\frac{1}{2}$ times annual salary, and for younger members the amount was one times annual salary ('annual salary' for GPs is defined as average annual dynamized remuneration).

2 Death benefit for scheme members with preserved pensions is three times pension, the better of the two options previously available.

This simplifies rather than improves the situation; no member is any worse off as a consequence.

3 A 'death deficiency payment' is sometimes payable following a death after retirement. This payment now guarantees an amount equal to five years' pension, subject to an overriding maximum payment of two times the level of annual salary

earned at the date of retirement minus the lump sum paid at retirement.

This is a substantial improvement, despite the limit on the total sum payable. For example, under the previous rules, if a male member on full pension died the day immediately following the date of retirement, his spouse would have received only a widow's pension and no further lump sum. Under the new proposals, an additional lump sum equal to 50% of annual salary would also be payable. This is shown by the following example:

	£
Salary at retirement	50 000
Pension ($\frac{40}{80}$ ths)	25 000
Lump sum at retirement (three times pension)	75 000
Death deficiency payment	
= 5 × pension = 5 × £25 000	125 000
But	
Overriding maximum	
= 2 × annual salary = 2 × £50 000	100 000
less retirement lump sum	75 000
	£25 000

The spouse receives the maximum sum of £25 000.

4   Voluntary early retirement can now be taken from the age of 50 with actuarially reduced benefits.

This new provision means that members can now choose to retire before the age of 60 and take their pension and lump sum. Previously, this option was only available to individuals retiring because of ill health, redundancy, organizational change, in the interests of the service or under the 'achieving a balance' arrangements, or to those with special class/mental health officer (MHO) status.

The pension and lump sum accrued up until retirement date are actuarially reduced to take account of the effects of paying these before the normal retirement age of 60. The actuarial reduction is calculated as shown in Table 16.1.

Thus, someone retiring at the age of 58 would receive 89% of the

Table 16.1 Voluntary early retirement: calculating the actuarial reduction

Age	Proportion of the amount accrued by that age	
	Pension	Lump sum
50	0.599	0.747
51	0.624	0.769
52	0.652	0.792
53	0.682	0.815
54	0.716	0.839
55	0.754	0.864
56	0.796	0.889
57	0.841	0.916
58	0.890	0.943
59	0.943	0.971

pension accrued by the age of 58, *rather than 60*. Similarly, the lump sum would be 94.3% of that lump sum accrued by the age of 58.

Appendix B gives details of the actuarial reduction based on completed years and months.

Similar levels of reduction are also used in private and other public sector pension schemes if a pension is drawn before normal retiring age.

5   **In certain circumstances, it will be possible to take voluntary early retirement from the age of 50 without any actuarial reduction but with no enhancement of benefits such as those paid for other types of early retirement. However, this is subject to the discretion of local management, who must meet the extra cost involved.**

The employer must meet the cost of the pension from the date of retirement up to the normal retirement age of 60, as well as the extra cost of paying the lump sum before normal retirement age.

Early retirement without actuarial reduction is not available to GPs. As they are self-employed, there is no local management able to exercise the necessary discretionary powers and meet the cost. However, the General Medical Services Committee of the BMA is pursuing with the Health Department possible ways of extending this provision to GPs.

These new early retirement arrangements are voluntary – they cannot be used to retire staff compulsorily – nor do they replace existing early retirement arrangements that provide for *enhanced* pension and lump sum. Those facing circumstances in which one of the following options may be appropriate should take particular care to ensure that they are being offered the correct early retirement package (which should usually provide enhanced benefits):

- ill health

- redundancy

- organizational change

- in the interests of the service

- 'achieving a balance'.

Care also needs to be taken by anyone with special class or MHO status. Staff in these categories can retire on full pension at the age of 55. However, if they retire before then, they automatically lose their special status under the new early retirement provisions, and the same actuarial reduction factors will be applied to them as any other scheme member. For example, if they retire at 54, they will receive only 71.6% of the pension accrued at that age, whereas by waiting just one further year they would have received 100% of pension accrued at the age of 55.

Members taking voluntary early retirement cannot rejoin the NHS pension scheme if they subsequently return to NHS work. However, a pension can be built up in the new job through a personal pension plan.

Although abatement has been abolished for those aged 60 and over (see below), members who take voluntary early retirement will be subject to abatement (see Chapter 15) if they return to work before this age.

Scheme members who opt for early retirement before the age of 55 need to note that their pension is not inflation proofed until the age of 55. However, at this point, there is a 'catching-up' exercise to cover inflation increases in the period since retirement.

6   **The NHS ill-health pension can now be commuted into a lump sum if a member is terminally ill. Terminal illness is defined as a life expectancy of less than 12 months. The benefit paid is a tax-free lump sum of five times the ill-health pension, subject to an overriding cap equal to two times pay minus the retirement lump sum. The normal retirement lump sum is also payable. There is no reduction in either figure in respect of pre-1972 service.**

The commuted lump sum will be reduced by the amount of guaranteed minimum pension payable: this is non-commutable and is that element of the NHS pension (and other occupational pensions) that must be paid under State pension legislation.

Dependants' benefits will continue to be paid in full.

7 Retirement arrangements after the normal NHS retirement age of 60 have been changed so that:

- members can choose their retirement date, rather than have benefits automatically paid when a particular post ends after the age of 60, as was previously the case even if a concurrent post was continuing

- retirement (which will result in payment of pension and lump sum) must involve a significant break in employment before any return to work.

8 At retirement, NHS pension scheme membership ends permanently. However, if a member aged 60 or over returns to work in the NHS, the pension will not be abated.

The abolition of abatement, even with the following restrictions, represents a significant improvement. The restrictions are:

- abatement continues until the age of 60 for anyone who has retired before that age (whatever the reason for the early retirement)

- there must be a significant break (of at least one month) in employment before returning to work

- it is not possible to rejoin the NHS pension scheme and build up extra benefits after returning to NHS work (but see below).

Other features include the following:

- anyone retiring on ill-health grounds can rejoin the NHS pension scheme if they return to work before the age of 50

- although no-one else can rejoin the scheme, a personal pension plan can be used to build additional pension benefits

- the concept of 24-hour retirement has effectively gone; however, GPs can return to work after one month's break if partners, the FHSA or Health Board and medical practices committee agree

- if a member returns to work within one month, the pension is with-drawn completely until the new post ends. This is not the same as abatement, which only occurs if the total sum of post-retirement income and pension exceeds pre-retirement income

- it is not necessary to take a whole month's break (or, in fact, any break) from a continuing part-time post of less than 16 hours per week, although scheme membership, as such, must end for all posts

- once a retirement date has been selected, pension benefits have to be drawn in respect of all NHS posts, including any continuing part-time posts. The only exception is where a member is made redundant from one post while continuing in another; in these circumstances, there is a choice between taking benefits based on all service so far and ending scheme membership completely, or taking benefit for the redundant post only and continuing scheme membership

- the abatement rules for those still subject to them are eased by allowing annual assessment

- members who have two or more posts with different salaries can no longer retire from the higher-paid post first and have all previous service pensioned at its salary level. A composite salary is now used to calculate benefits accrued from all posts

- for anyone being abated on 6 March 1995, abatement will continue until they retire again, when they become subject to the new rules.

9   Modification of benefits has been abolished.

The term 'modification' refers to the fact that the NHS pension of some members was reduced by a small amount (usually £50 per annum or less) to take account of a period prior to 1980 when people paid a reduced or 'modified' contribution to their occupational pension schemes. This modified level was designed to ensure that contributions to an occupational pension scheme plus contributions to the State scheme did not, in total, exceed a certain level.

10   Early retirement arrangements that allowed female nurses, physiotherapists, health visitors and midwives to retire at the age of 55 (all having special class status) were extended from 17 May 1990 to include male staff in these categories. However, this special class status, and mental health officer

(MHO) status, have both been withdrawn for new entrants. Special class/MHO status is retained by those already holding it.

If male special class staff do retire at 55, the pension will only be based on service since 17 May 1990. Earlier service will be preserved for payment at age 60.

The withdrawal of special class/MHO status applies to new entrants only, but the status continues to be available to existing holders. Existing holders who subsequently give up the status will be able to regain it if they remain within the NHS pension scheme. If they leave the scheme, they can only regain it if they return to the scheme within five years. Those who lost the status before 6 March 1995 will also be able to regain it if they stay in the NHS scheme or if they return to the scheme within five years of leaving it.

Other changes to the NHS pension scheme.

GP practice staff

The government has, in principle, approved general medical practitioner practice staff entering the NHS pension scheme; however, it is not willing to proceed until the likely cost of this change has been assessed. The Health Department is undertaking a survey of the current staffing and pension arrangements of GP practices in order to enable the likely cost to be assessed. In addition, the Department will need to discuss the details of the proposed arrangements with the BMA's General Medical Services Committee. It seems unlikely that practice staff will be able to join the scheme before 1996, if in fact, the government does confirm that they can do so.

Additional voluntary contributions (AVCs)

Trust employers are able to make contributions to additional voluntary and free-standing additional voluntary contribution (AVC/FSAVC) plans on behalf of employees, so that they may build up additional pension benefits at no cost to themselves. The limits on benefits, explained in Chapter 5, remain the same, whether the contributor to the AVC/FSAVC plan is the employer or the employee.

Added years
The existing arrangements for purchasing added years will be reviewed, with the intention of making them more flexible and intelligible and examining ways of integrating them with the new voluntary early retirement arrangements.

17

State benefits on retirement

State basic pension • Additional pension (the State
Earnings-Related Pension – SERPS) • Graduated pension
• Widows and widowers • Divorce • Invalidity benefit
• Attendance allowance • State pension age for women
• Pensions forecast • Claiming your pension • Further
information

For most people retiring from the NHS, their main source of income in retirement will be their NHS pension. There should also be some invest-ment income from the lump sum if this is invested at retirement, and there may be additional pension from a personal pension plan (PPP).

For many, this income should be sufficient to ensure a satisfactory standard of living in retirement. However, the benefits available from the State should not be overlooked; this chapter outlines these.

State basic pension

The State basic pension for the year commencing 6 April 1995 is £58.85 per week for a single person. For a married couple, it depends upon whether the wife has paid full contributions; if she has, she may also receive £58.85. If not, she can receive £35.25, making a total of £94.10 for a married couple.

The pension is payable from age 65 for a man and age 60 for a woman; this age difference is expected to be abolished during the next decade or so.

Those women who opted to pay the married woman's reduced rate contribution can only be paid the lower rate of pension (£35.25), but it cannot be claimed until the husband reaches age 65. If the woman is under 60 when her husband turns 65, he can claim on her behalf an 'adult dependency allowance', which is the same as the married woman's pension (£35.25). This is means tested until payable as a right to the woman at the age of 60.

The State basic pension is index linked: it is increased each year in line with the retail prices index. It is payable if the pensioner is living overseas (and can be paid anywhere), but in this case may not be index linked unless there is a reciprocal agreement with the country concerned. Anyone thinking of retiring to an overseas country should seek advice from their local Department of Social Security office before departure.

Who qualifies for the State basic pension?

Whether you receive the pension, and, if so, how much you receive, depends upon your national insurance contributions. To receive the full pension, you need to contribute for about 90% of your working life. For national insurance purposes, a working life is 49 years for a man (from 16–65 years old) and 44 years (16–60) for a woman.

However, there are five 'free' years, so that a full contribution record is actually 44 years for a man and 39 years for a woman. In addition, if not working, a man is automatically credited with the years from age 60–65, so that he effectively needs 39 working years in total. If the man works between the ages 60 and 65, he must continue to pay national insurance contributions. Beyond State pension age, contributions do not have to be paid. Years of full-time education between the ages of 16 and 18 are also automatically credited, but not the years of full-time education after the age of 18 (which is, of course, of relevance to doctors, who are usually in full-time education until the age of at least 23).

In addition, credits are given for any periods of claiming certain State benefits, including unemployment, maternity and sickness benefits. Anyone retiring before age 60 may wish to register as unemployed in order to ensure continuing credits of national insurance contributions (even if unemployment benefit is not payable because the NHS pension has commenced).

All NHS employees are liable for Class 1 national insurance contributions. GPs, as self-employed contractors, are liable for Class 2 contributions plus Class 4 contributions relating to profits.

It can be difficult to achieve a full contribution record and therefore to qualify for the full pension. Doctors, for instance, are disadvantaged by not qualifying until the age of at least 23. It is possible to pay voluntary contributions in order to make up for lost years as a student or periods spent overseas but very few people do so and it is only possible to make such extra payments within six years of the 'lost' period concerned.

Women are, of course, disadvantaged by any career breaks they may take in having children and raising a family. However, Home Responsibilities Protection provides some help in this case.

Home Responsibilities Protection (HRP)
HRP, which was introduced in 1978, reduces the years of national insurance credits needed to qualify for a pension, as shown in the example below. (It is assumed in this case that the woman qualifies for 12 HRP years.)

	Years
Potential working life	44
less five 'free' years	5
Years needed for full pension	39
less HRP years	12
Working years needed for full pension	27

HRP can apply in the following cases:

- if you are the 'main payee' for child benefit for a child under age 16 *or*

- if you receive income support in order to care for someone at home *or*

- if you are looking after someone who receives attendance allowance.

Additional pension (the State Earnings-Related Pension – SERPS)

The SERPS pension (introduced in 1978) supplements the State basic pension and is based upon a complicated formula related to earnings. It can result in an extra pension of 25% of earnings between a lower and an upper earnings limit. This will reduce to 20% by the year 2010.

In common with most occupational pension schemes, the NHS pension scheme is contracted out of SERPS. This means that NHS pension scheme members will not receive the SERPS pension. Instead, they receive at least the guaranteed minimum pension (GMP), which is roughly the same as would have been payable under SERPS. Of course, in most cases, the NHS scheme pension is far greater than the GMP.

Because the NHS scheme is contracted out of SERPS, its members pay a substantially reduced rate of national insurance contributions; the amount of the reduction is currently 1.8% of salary.

Graduated pension

The Graduated Retirement Pension Scheme was an earnings-related scheme lasting from 1961 to 1975. This produces a small additional pension, no more than £5 or £6 per week. The Pensions Forecast Unit will let you have the exact figure if you send them form BR19 (see below).

Widows and Widowers

Widows

A widow's pension may be payable from the age of 45, and at the age of 60 there is an option to switch to the State basic pension, which can be up to a maximum for a single person, based on the husband's contributions and/or the widow's own contributions. There is no widow's pension payable from SERPS for widows of NHS pensioners because the NHS pension scheme provides a widow's pension at least equivalent to the SERPS entitlement. A widow receives half the husband's graduated pension.

Widowers

It may be possible to take the wife's contributions into account if this produces a better State pension for the widower, up to the maximum pension for a single person. The NHS pension scheme will provide a widower's pension equivalent to the SERPS entitlement. Half the wife's graduated pension is payable to the widower.

Divorce

People who are divorced may be able to use some of the national insurance credits of a former spouse to increase the amount of State basic pension payable. There is no entitlement to part of the former spouse's SERPS or graduated pension.

Invalidity benefit

Invalidity benefit may be payable if a person is incapable of work because of sickness or disability. This may be applicable, for instance, if an NHS pension scheme member has retired on the grounds of ill health and/or is in receipt of NHS injury benefit. Once State retirement age (60 for women and 65 for men) has been reached, there is an option to switch from invalidity benefit to the State basic pension, which is calculated in a similar way. From the age of 65 (women) and 70 (men), the State pension must be paid instead.

From April 1995 invalidity benefit (and sickness benefit) is to be replaced by incapacity benefit.

Attendance allowance

Some people approaching retirement will be caring for elderly or infirm relatives and may be able to obtain an attendance allowance. This is not usually means tested.

State pension age for women

The government has announced that State pension ages are to be equalized by raising the age for women from 60 to 65. This change will be phased in between the years 2010 and 2020. Women born before 6 April 1950 will not be affected, retaining their right to a State pension at the age of 60.

The phased introduction affects women born between 6 April 1950 and 5 April 1955. They will receive a pension at an age of 60 plus one month for every month their birthday falls after 5 April 1950; for example, someone born in October 1950 would receive a State pension at 60 years 7 months old. Women born after 5 April 1955 will receive the pension at the age of 65.

Pensions forecast

You can find out what your State pension is likely to be by obtaining a pensions forecast form (BR19) from your local social security office and sending this off to the Pensions Forecast Unit in Newcastle.

Claiming your pension

You should receive a claim form before your State pension age; if this does not arrive, contact your local social security office.

Further information

Details of the full range of State benefits can be obtained from your local Benefits Agency or Department of Social Security office. They also produce a number of easy-to-read leaflets, including 'Benefits after Retirement' (FB32) and 'A Guide to Retirement Pensions' (NP46).

There are also some useful telephone numbers to keep in mind; calls are free and the staff are helpful:

0800 666555   Freeline social security is a general information service on all aspects of social security and national insurance.

Freeline social security is also available in four other languages:

Chinese	0800 252451
Punjabi	0800 521360
Urdu	0800 289188
Welsh	0800 289011

0800 882200   This is the benefit enquiry line, providing advice to disabled people and their carers.

0800 393539   This is a line for employers; it may be useful for GPs and practice managers as it provides general advice and information about national insurance contributions and employer-paid benefits.

18

Pensions in a changing society

Demographic and social changes since 1947 • Divorce
• Women at work • Unmarried partners • One-parent
families • Job mobility • Married working couples

Since the NHS pension scheme was established in 1947, there have been
far-reaching social and economic changes. The NHS pension scheme, in
common with other occupational pension schemes, has failed to keep pace
with those changes. This chapter discusses some of the issues involved and
their impact upon NHS staff, their partners and their families.

When new public sector occupational schemes were being established
following the Second World War, it was generally assumed that the man
would be the breadwinner and that his wife (and children) would be
provided for in retirement by means of his pension. It was assumed that
marriages would normally last to retirement and beyond, unless death
intervened.

The basic framework of most occupational pension schemes is still
based on these traditional assumptions. There is a pension of up to 50%
of salary (or effectively two-thirds of salary if the lump sum is taken into
account) and a widow's pension of 50% of this, together with provision
for up to two children. Indeed, the whole scheme is built around the
archetypal nuclear family, comprising husband, wife and two children (the
only departure from this stereotype being that there is no requirement
for the two children to be of different sexes!). Unfortunately, the nuclear
family (which was always somewhat mythical) is now an endangered
species.

Demographic and social changes since 1947

The pattern of family life has changed substantially since 1947:

• women are much more likely to have their own careers and pensions.

In 1992, women comprised 52% of the intake into medical and dental schools

- one in two marriages is ending in divorce. The proportion is even higher among second marriages

- a smaller proportion of the population is getting married: there were 13% fewer marriages in 1991 than in 1981

- people are more likely to cohabit and procreate without marrying

- there has been a large increase in the proportion of one-parent families

- homosexuality has been legalized, and it is not unusual for partners of the same sex to establish long-term relationships

- increased life expectancy has raised the importance of planning for retirement.

These complex, and sometimes controversial, changes are having a major impact on pensions and retirement, as is explained below.

Divorce

A divorced partner has no entitlement within the NHS pension scheme. This has created major problems now that the divorce rate has reached such high levels. A woman marrying in the late 1940s or 1950s could have expected her husband's pension to provide for her in retirement. During the intervening years, she is likely to have provided invaluable support to her husband in his own career, taking the major responsibility for home and family. Yet, she will receive nothing from his pension scheme if he dies after they have divorced. Moreover, if the couple divorce late in his career, she will have had no opportunity to build up a pension in her own right. To add insult to injury, if the husband remarries shortly before he retires, his new wife will be eligible to receive a full widow's pension. Even if he remarries after retirement, the new wife will still be eligible for a widow's pension, albeit one which is based on his service since 1978 only.

The blatant inequity of these pension arrangements is widely recognized, and it is generally accepted that reform is long overdue. However, there are some crucial legal and technical matters that need to be resolved.

The Pensions Management Institute and the Law Society appointed a joint working group to examine the issue of pensions and divorce. Its report, published in 1993, recommended that provision should be made at the time of divorce to ensure that the value of the working partner's pension is taken into account in the divorce settlement and that part of it is transferred to the divorced spouse. It was hoped that the government's 1994 White Paper on pensions would address this issue. However, the government proposed only that additional research should be carried out, with a view to looking at the question again, perhaps towards the end of 1995.

Women at work

Recent European Court judgements have established that it is illegal to discriminate on the basis of gender in respect of pension provision. Unfortunately, these judgements have also established that equality does not have to be retrospective (except that part-timers can now claim pension scheme membership back to 1976). For example, in the NHS pension scheme, widowers' pensions were introduced for the first time in 1988; if a woman dies before her husband, he will receive a pension based only on her service since that year. However, if a man dies before his wife, a widow's pension is paid based on full service pre- and post-1988. Thus, women members of the scheme have substantially inferior insurance cover for their families, despite the fact that they have always paid the same contribution rates as men.

Many women find it difficult to accumulate maximum pension benefits because of the need to combine family commitments with their careers. NHS pension scheme benefits are dependent upon length of service and income, and any breaks in service, because of family commitments or any other reason, can have a significant impact on the final value of these benefits:

- a break in service of over 12 months within two years of joining the scheme results in a refund of contributions
- any break results in a reduced service credit
- part-time working results in reduced benefits.

Furthermore, if the break limits the woman's career progress, her final pension will be based on a lower final salary than would otherwise have been the case.

For women GPs, any GP locum work or work within the retainer scheme is not superannuable, and employment as a salaried assistant is not necessarily superannuable. Furthermore, because a career break inevitably slows down progress towards a full share of partnership profits, this also adversely affects final pension (GPs' pensions being based on total superannuable income earned throughout their careers).

Job sharing also results in a reduced pension. In this case, salaried doctors' pensionable service only accrues at a part-time rate, and GPs' pensions are reduced in proportion to the lower income resulting from the job share.

It is possible to acquire extra benefits by paying additional contributions, but the extent to which this alleviates the difficulties outlined above is limited.

Unmarried partners

The dramatic increase in divorce has been accompanied by a substantial rise in the number of people living together outside marriage. Moreover, many people choose not to marry, even though they may establish a permanent relationship. The NHS pension scheme pays a spouse's pension only to a legally married husband or wife. Unmarried partners without separate pension provision therefore face serious financial difficulties if their partner dies before them. They do not receive a pension, either the normal spouse's pension payable if someone dies after retirement or the enhanced pension payable on death in service. Also, access to the lump sum is not automatic. This will be paid into the deceased person's estate, and the partner will only receive it if named in a properly drawn-up will. Partners of the same sex face similar disadvantages.

Fortunately, children's allowances are payable even if the parents were not married.

Unlike the NHS pension scheme, some other pension schemes have formally recognized unmarried partners. They allow any member without a spouse to nominate an adult dependant to receive the pension where there is no spouse. However, the scope for this improved arrangement is limited because the Inland Revenue insists on a 'dependency' test. This means that the pension is not payable to the nominated partner as of right but can only be paid if the partner was genuinely financially dependent upon the deceased member.

It is possible for NHS scheme members to give up part of their pension and to 'allocate' this to an unmarried partner if the partner is dependent upon them (see Chapter 8).

One-parent families

The growth in the number of one-parent families has been widely publicized and has attracted considerable political controversy. It is another consequence of the breakdown of the traditional family structure within the UK, a concept on which the NHS pension scheme and other occupational pension schemes have always been based.

If the single parent divorces an NHS pension scheme member, or is a member of the NHS pension scheme but only able to work part-time, or needs a career break, there are serious implications for pension and subsequent income in retirement.

Job mobility

There is general expectation that people are (or should be) more mobile during their careers, moving more frequently between occupations, jobs and employers. Indeed, they often have mobility forced upon them by redundancy or greatly reduced career opportunities.

The NHS pension scheme and other pension schemes are not designed to accommodate this phenomenon satisfactorily. The traditional years of service/final salary scheme only fully rewards the person who stays and makes an entire career with the same employer and, conversely, usually penalizes the early leaver. Although it is possible to transfer benefits between schemes, service credit is often lost on transfer. Consequently, anyone moving between several employers during their career is likely to end up with substantially lower pension benefits.

If accumulated benefits are left in the NHS pension scheme, they are increased in line with inflation, a better arrangement than in the private sector, in which most schemes only increase preserved pensions by the statutory maximum of 5% per annum (or the inflation rate, if lower). In any case, salary increases are generally greater than the rate of inflation, and the eventual pension earned over a given period will be less than if the person had not left the NHS.

Insurance benefits within pension schemes are also at risk when moving between jobs. The scheme receiving the new member normally lays down a waiting period before he or she becomes eligible for certain benefits. The NHS scheme's waiting period for enhanced benefits is five years. Indeed, *preserved* benefits in the NHS pension scheme are not enhanced even if the former member dies, or is unable to work and an ill-health pension is payable.

Even job mobility within the NHS can reduce pension entitlement. For example, a doctor moving between practitioner and non-practitioner work may receive a reduced pension as a result, even though the NHS encourages such mobility.

Married working couples

Although most of the changes discussed above lead to a number of pitfalls in the pension field, there is one area in which people may actually be accumulating more pension than they need.

Married couples, at least those choosing not to have children, may well build up full pensions in their own pension schemes plus provision for a full spouse's pension to be payable on their death. The surviving spouse could therefore have a pension in his or her own right equal to two-thirds final salary, plus a spouse's pension of half of their partner's full pension. Taking the State pension into account as well, a person in this position may have a retirement income in excess of their salary when working. This certainly looks like over-provision, particularly in view of the fact that outgoings tend to be reduced after retirement.

19

Health

DAVID WELLS

Exercise • Diet • Alcohol • Smoking

May I offer you some light relief from all these slightly dull but important facts and figures and give you some of my personal thoughts on health? I will speak from the point of view of 30 years in general practice, with the wisdom gained from the great privilege of being alongside many hundreds of people at their times of crisis, and from five years' retirement of my own. Medicine is a mixture of science and art, and as you all have access to the science via your GP, let me concentrate more on the art of healthy living.

First, let me suggest what I hope will be a helpful way of looking at yourself in relation to the maintenance of health. Imagine an apothecary's balance with its two scales, with one labelled 'physical' and the other 'mental'. This reminds us that a proper balance between physical and mental activities is vital to our health. By now you should all have got a very good idea of what sort of balance suits your own make-up, even if you seldom achieve it. Remember that, from now on, it may be more difficult to blame anyone else for any imbalance. Imagine now the cross-bar of the balance with the pivot being as frictionless as possible, and let's label this 'social'. This reminds us that people and relationships are also of great importance to our well-being and that the less friction there is here, the better. Imagine now the base of the balance, which needs to be firm and sound for the instrument to do its job properly; let's call this 'spiritual', using its broadest and non-denominational definition. Out attitudes, priorities and beliefs are here and, as well as affecting our lifestyles, I believe they will also make a fundamental difference to our general bodily functions. Think of the long-standing, right-sided abdominal pain cured overnight by the removal of the fear of appendicitis or cancer that was quite reasonably maintaining the pain. Think of the pain-wracked person admitted to a hospice, where the pain is relieved by being treated as a whole and valued person and often a smaller dose of analgesic than before, with much greater effect. Think of the ME sufferer given a purely physical explanation of his complaint and his often depressingly slow progress, compared with the sometimes quite rapid recovery of the person who can be helped to tackle things on the triple platform of Body, Mind and Spirit. Even cardiac surgeons know the importance of a thorough overall preparation of their patients before surgery, in relation to the speed and degree of their recovery.

Let me now turn from the balance – but remember that a balance is essentially mobile and may need constant adjustment – to the topic of awareness. Old car enthusiasts, of which I am one, will know that you need to keep a constant ear open for any new rattles and squeaks, as well as keeping the seat of your pants sensitive to the ride and to any unusual vibration. Many of us may have spent much of our time positively ignoring messages from our bodies if they were inconvenient, often with dire results. Perhaps it is time for us to reassess our attitude to our bodies and to take more active notice of its messages to us. How about Jesus' Second Commandment, where He tells us to love our neighbours as we love ourselves. Any parent or grandparent amongst you will know the fundamental difference between loving and liking someone (unless my children are quite different from yours).

We need to enjoy and care for the amazing piece of equipment that has been given us, with the responsibility of reporting any untoward change in its working. My old Triumph Herald needs the expert attention of Ian the mechanic when it has a problem, but let us not forget that our bodies have a built-in repair and recovery mechanism as part of the original design, and that most of our medicines and ministrations are designed to help and encourage this innate recovery process, rather than working on their own.

So what do we do when some symptom requires us to take action? Remember that general practice is essentially personal doctoring and that half the responsibility for this relationship is our own, to ensure good communication and hence good personal advice being given to us. Our own GP is there to help us plot our course through any illness episode, assist where possible, and essentially offer us individual advice and guidance. For our own part, we need to know how our particular practice functions, so we need to have obtained, and to have read, our own practice's booklets (did anyone say 'What are they?'). The better we understand the practice, the better value we can get from it, for be assured that the health service is likely to continue to be under severe pressure for the rest of your life and mine.

Nearly all medical conditions are treatable, that is helpable rather than curable, and our GP will, by and large, give us as much help as we need, providing we tell him or her as clearly as possible how we are feeling and what we actually want. For example, do we just want reassurance that something is OK or are we after some treatment for it because we don't want to put up with it any more? Please don't be afraid of telling the receptionist something of your problem or needs, because it will almost certainly help her to successfully squeeze a quart into a pint pot.

If you have a problem or question, go to your own practice. However, these are a few general points I would like to make. Remember that although your complaint may have some connection with 'your age', please don't equate this with 'you must put up with it'. Most things are indeed treatable.

As you get older, your skin is likely to become drier, which is not healthy for it, so be prepared to use a moisturizing cream rather than waiting for a problem to develop.

Loss of hearing is potentially a very isolating condition, so when *all* of your friends have started to mumble, consider a hearing aid before you really have to have it – and keep your friends.

There are two sorts of depression – gloom and an anxiety–depressive illness. Gloom will pass, but the illness needs treatment, which is usually very effective. The illness is briefly characterized by unusually early waking – often about 2 am – and depression that is out of proportion, both in time and degree. Please consult your GP on behalf of yourself, your spouse or your friend, but also be aware that 'anti-depressants' do not treat gloom but only the anxiety–depressive illness.

Cancer is normally painless in its early stage, so don't wait for something to hurt before seeking advice.

Please understand that insomnia, or not sleeping very long, will not do you any real harm, excluding sleep deprivation such as from a visit of the younger grandchildren. You may not like it, but sleep patterns do change, so if you do end up with a sleeping tablet, you must ask yourself not 'Did I sleep longer?' but 'Do I feel any better?' Generally speaking, people do not feel better after sleeping medication if they can accept that they will come to no harm. The 'Mediterranean' siesta may be worth considering now we are all European.

Memory can be a problem at any stage, but as we age, it is the short-term memory that goes first. One way of by-passing some of the difficulties that can arise is to establish some habits – obsessionally, if you like – in relation to where important things, such as credit cards, car keys, cheque books and purse, are kept. If the habit becomes sufficiently ingrained, guess where the objects are when we have 'lost' them?

Hoping that your retirement may include some travel, especially by air, dehydration can present one of the major sources of fatigue and strain. Particularly in pressurized airliners, drink plenty and regularly during the journey, but remember that alcohol, particularly spirits, is actually dehydrating, so concentrate on 'Adam's ale'.

Exercise

Most of us have a mental picture of an elderly person, either true or fictitious, that may or may not equate with the road sign 'Elderly crossing', with two stooping and stick-wielding people. All the conditions we associate with old age can, interestingly, be divided roughly down the middle, half being due to various diseases (which probably increases statistically with the passage of years) and the other half being due to, guess what? – inactivity! 'Use it or lose it' has a great deal of truth in it, as shown by the fact that loss of strength with increasing age is more to do with laziness or delegating physical activities to others, rather than just the passage of years. This means that activity is really not an optional extra, but if we do want to crumble, then just sit quietly and wait; it may not be long. If we don't enjoy an activity, we won't do it, so we must all find physical activities that we can enjoy (if we don't already have them). Remember that group activities can often encourage us to join in when individually we may well not want to bother, be it an actual sporting occasion or a communal activity. For non-sporting members, can I reassure you that in my experience the most important attribute is a positive attitude to life, which leads on to all sorts of activities and exercise, rather than just the actual exercise. Whatever it is going to be for you – **do it**. If it can be something that exercises body, mind and spirit in one activity, so much the better.

Diet

This is a fascinating subject, because when you look critically at all the information around, nearly all of it is either theory or pure statistics, with very few facts or real accepted understanding of diet. So pay your money and take your choice, but let me offer a few generally agreed points. We were constructed to have two or three regular, smallish meals, rather than one large one.

Dehydration is increasingly deleterious to health as we age. The best general indicator is our bowels, where a small, hard stool (constipation) shows a lack of fluid in the body, so we need to take in more fluid, as well as probably increasing our fibre intake to hold the fluid in the body.

We know that too much salt puts about half the population into heart failure as we age, so make sure you are not having more than you really want – and please taste your food before you put salt on (with apologies to those with shares in salt companies). We also know that animal fat is not good for us in a variety of ways, so, again, do with as little as you can reasonably manage; however, fish and vegetable fats are generally good for us. Currently, we seem, as a nation, to be eating more fish and less meat.

Sugar is a very concentrated form of energy and appears to be bad for us in a number of ways, so, as before, do with as little as you can manage. Eating is fun, so enjoy it. A lot is habit, so consider keeping a good balance in both quantity (being overweight *is* bad for health, I'm afraid) and quality on a day-to-day basis. At any family occasion, eat what you like; it won't do any harm. What your own body is telling you, if you listen carefully, is of more useful guidance to you than any advice from outside.

Alcohol

Sorry folks, alcohol is a poison. This is a fact, not opinion. But every cloud has a silver lining, and part of God's original design for us is a very effective detoxicating unit – our liver – which will remove one unit of alcohol in one hour if it is working well. Any book on alcohol will give you a table of what quantity is safe, but let me warn you they are all based on other people's livers. How is your own liver? Don't rely on blood tests; when you have taken poison (yes, I know, it is pleasant) ask yourself how you feel the next morning and wait for an honest answer. Some people may find that one unit is their limit, others may find that they can manage much more on occasions, but if you don't feel well, it may well be that you haven't processed the poison, in which case you must refrain until the body is fully recovered. There are many statistics that suggest that moderate drinking, such as a daily whisky or glass of red wine, is good for you, and that it will protect you from this, that and the other. My personal opinion is that a poison can't possibly do you any good, but moderate, sensible drinking is evidence of a moderate, sensible, balanced sort of life style, and that the beneficial part of the equation is the life style rather than the alcohol. A little of what you fancy does you good!

Smoking

The problems associated with smoking have changed fundamentally in the past few years, because of its changed public health aspect. It is now legally accepted that the lung problems of smoking also apply to passive smoking, and I am sure that more and more public places will go 'non-smoking'. We all remember the jumbo jet that crashed at Lockerbie some years ago, but do we all understand that two jumbo-jets-worth of people every week die from smoking-related illness. Think of the economics, let alone the suffering, involved. Smoking seriously increases the risk of heart disease, but within about six to eight months of stopping, the risks have reverted to the non-smoking rate, so it is never too late to give up. We know for certain that smoking interferes with the oxygen supply to the developing baby in the uterus, and it is reasonably clear that it interferes in some way with our immune system – the defence and repair department – although it is a sedative, and a very rapidly acting one at that. I don't believe we can tell our own young not to smoke, unless, as the grand-parental generation, we set them a good example. Do we still really need a 'sedative', I wonder, in retirement?

Retirement is a time of change, both the obvious and the quite subtle, and this applies to spouses as well. From the health point of view, there are two important areas to consider. The first is our relationships around the home. The general timetable at home is going to change, so there is an opportunity to plan for time to work on our relationships, if we admit that they could do with it. One of the quicker ways of damaging your health is to have a sour relationship on the go – and remember that half of the responsibility for that relationship is on your shoulders, so please think about it. The other aspect to be considered is the fact that we leave our labels behind when we stop work, which gives us the opportunity to become more fully our real selves. We have the opportunity to reassess our identity or status and to consider whether it relates to what others think of us or of how we see ourselves. Going back to Jesus' Second Commandment, and about loving being all about acceptance, we must accept ourselves as we are, abilities and disabilities together, and then take an active and positive approach to the next chapter of our lives.

I think most of us want to make the best of our health, realizing that we are neither immortal nor invincible. Thinking of the balance concept I started with, I submit that our best bet is to concentrate on keeping the balance steady as our circumstances change over the course of time. I suspect we all know people who may have quite severe disabilities but who have somehow kept the balance steady, as well as others who have no disease process apparent but are 'unbalanced' and 'unhealthy'. So much more responsibility and opportunity is in our own hands than we often realize, so let's go out and make the best of our health opportunities.

20

Leisure in retirement

Social activities • Physical activities • Intellectual activities • Spiritual well-being

On retirement, an enormous amount of time suddenly becomes available. For most people, this will the greatest availability of free time since their childhood, and for the first time in their lives, they will be genuinely free to choose how to make use of it.

At least 2000 extra hours per year become available when someone retires, a figure that only takes account of average working hours and commuting time. The figure is obviously far higher for many NHS workers, who may work far longer than average hours, take fewer holidays or make long journeys to work. It is much higher again if one takes into account the many hours spent at home preparing for work or recovering from the fatigue and stress caused by work.

Of course, this free time presents an attractive opportunity for rest and fulfilment, but it is often not grasped as it should be and can so easily be squandered unless thought and preparation is given to its best use. Indeed, its sudden availability is a challenge as much as it is an opportunity.

We have all worked with colleagues who have been so engrossed in their work that when they retire we ask how they can possibly cope with the loss of their work. What will they do with their time? Fortunately, most of us also know other retired colleagues who are so busy, and happily busy, that they cannot imagine how they ever found time to go to work!

There is, of course, no perfect way of ensuring a happy retirement. Finance and health play a large part, as do an individual's personality and experience prior to retirement age. Nevertheless, for most people, there are wonderful opportunities available, which can make the retirement years the most fulfilling and happy of all.

It is said that it is best to have an indoor activity and an outdoor one, a physical pursuit and an intellectual one, a time alone and a time with people. There is little doubt that the question of balance is important for good health and for a good retirement.

This chapter divides leisure activities into the four general areas listed below (obviously with considerable overlap between them) and provides a brief overview to encourage further thought and discussion:

- social

- physical

- intellectual

- spiritual.

Social activities

Contact with people is a basic human need: we all need other people, in a variety of different ways. At retirement, a potential pitfall looms, in that our most frequent source of contact with people disappears and the danger of isolation arises. For almost everyone working in the NHS, the change is quite dramatic, because of the extensive contact with people that is an important part of NHS work. This change needs to be thought about and prepared for. It does not simply amount to no longer having contact with patients (a few of whom may be very easy to leave behind!) and colleagues at the work-place. Most people also see some of their colleagues socially, and there is a danger that this important contact ends completely or is greatly reduced at retirement. Retiring from work should not necessarily mean losing contact with friends who are still working.

Family and friends

Fortunately, one of the bonuses of retirement is that it offers increased time and opportunity to see other people, including family and friends. Many retired people have grandchildren who love to see them and value their experience and wisdom. Of course, this may have drawbacks, particularly if both parents work and grandparents are seen as potential long-term babysitters. This may be enjoyable for those who wish to spend leisure time in this way, but for others there will be a need to lay down ground rules so that babysitting duties are arranged on their terms and not necessarily on those of the parents.

Community activities

Contact with people might also come from activities within the local community. There are many possibilities including voluntary work (see Chapter 15), religious activities, clubs, political parties and pressure groups, etc. Retirement provides an opportunity to participate in an organization for which one feels an affinity and to an extent that one feels comfortable with.

Travel

Opportunities for travel have greatly expanded. Retired people have a big advantage in that they can travel off season and take advantage of price reductions and concessionary fares. Off-season travel has the added advantage of avoiding the crowds and the unpleasant congestion at airports and elsewhere.

Retired people constitute a continually expanding market, and major tour operators are already responding to this; SAGA Holidays (see Appendix A) is one example of a company specializing in holidays for the over 60s. Details of special holidays designed for retired people can be obtained from most travel agents.

Special interest holidays cater for a wide range of tastes, for example languages, art appreciation, architecture, walking, cycling, wine tasting and historical visits.

Opportunities have improved also for disabled people, and many travel agents help with their travel arrangements and accommodation. Some useful publications for the disabled traveller are listed in Appendix A.

British Rail offers excellent concessions to the over 60s, particularly the Senior Railcard, which gives a one-third discount. Senior citizens are almost always able to obtain concessions on buses, and there are often reduced fares available on coaches and airlines.

Physical activities

The human body ages in a physical sense less quickly than many people realize. In fact, for many people, retirement results in an immediate improvement in physical well-being and increased physical activity.

Maintaining physical fitness is, of course, important for good health but does not need to be a chore. On the contrary, the increased time available for gardening, walking, cycling, yoga, tennis, golf, swimming or keep fit classes is one of the great opportunities and pleasures of retirement. For many, this will be a continuation or extension of an enjoyable activity already experienced; for others, it may be a new opportunity to improve the quality of life.

Intellectual activities

For many people at work leading busy lives, the local library is a place visited rarely, if at all. Retirement offers the opportunity to use the libraries to rediscover the joys of reading and also as a source of much information about local, and not so local, groups and activities.

Many people have dabbled in other languages during their working lives, perhaps frustrated by the lack of time and energy needed to become more fluent. Language classes are widely available from adult education institutes, which can be supplemented by tapes and books. There is great pleasure to be gained from visiting a foreign country equipped with even just a little of the language.

Retirement offers the opportunity to visit the cinema and theatre often at prices, and certainly at times, not available to people at work. For lovers of music, there is the potential for concert-going, to join a choir or perhaps even to learn a favourite musical instrument. In fact, there are many musical, drama, artistic and crafts events throughout the country, often offering concessions to retired people.

People have an extraordinary range of hobbies, interests and skills, and there are many more to be discovered. Adult education institutes are especially useful for taking up a new intellectual, artistic or physical pursuit or improving an existing skill. Local libraries can provide details, and Londoners can purchase the publication 'Floodlight' from bookstalls.

The University of the Third Age offers a wide range of educational and leisure activities, and the Open University offer degrees and short courses for all ages (see Appendix A).

Spiritual well-being

Work plays such an important part in our lives that its loss can be hard to replace. The respect and affection of one's patients and colleagues can bring a sense of self-esteem and well-being that may need to be acquired in other ways in retirement. To feel good about oneself and at relative ease with the world is a very personal thing, not always easy to achieve, and will be acquired in different ways by different people.

People often welcome the opportunity that retirement brings to spend more time participating in the activities of their local place of worship, bringing spiritual well-being in a religious sense.

However, other avenues might be considered. The loss of a role and a sense of value and status may be overcome by working with a local group, club or charity, perhaps taking on a role such as secretary or treasurer, using skills acquired during one's working life, or even developing new skills as part of a reinvigorated life.

A sense of spiritual well-being may also be developed in other ways, by having the time and opportunity for activities such as meditation, yoga, reading or the pursuit of a favourite hobby or activity.

21

Preparing for retirement

> Finance • Housing • Your partner • Caring for elderly
> parents • Health • Pre-retirement courses

In one sense, preparing for retirement begins very early in life. It is never too soon to start a pension, organize finances carefully, begin looking after long-term health or develop interests outside one's work. Nevertheless, as retirement approaches, there is an opportunity to prepare for it in a number of specific and useful ways to help with what can be a difficult transition.

Finance

NHS pension scheme

The benefits of the NHS pension scheme are described in earlier chapters. As retirement approaches, it is a good idea to obtain an estimate of what your pension and lump sum are likely to be. This will not only make you aware of how much your main source of income will be in retirement, but may also help you to plan your date of retirement. Estimates can be obtained through your employer or FHSA/Health Board, or by writing directly to the relevant pensions agency (see Appendix A).

When obtaining an estimate, it is advisable to ask for a detailed service record. This enables you to check that all pensionable service has been properly recorded and taken into account in calculating your pension. Unfortunately, service records are not particularly reliable; mistakes and omissions can occur. This is particularly common if someone has had several employers during their career. Thus, doctors should take particular care to ensure that all posts have been recorded and that the correct dates and numbers of sessions are shown. Where there are mistakes or omissions, you should write to the pensions agency, which will investigate the service concerned and amend the service record.

GPs should ask not only for a service record but also for a complete dynamizing sheet. This will show superannuable income for every year, before and after it has been dynamized (see Chapter 3 for an explanation of dynamizing). It will also show how these years of income are totalled and the pension figure arrived at. The lump sum is also shown, including details of pre-1972 accrual if an unreduced lump sum has not been purchased.

It is advisable to resolve any queries about the service record or entitlements well before retirement. In fact, it is not too early to start planning several years before the intended retirement date.

It is worth remembering that easy-to-read guides on the NHS pension scheme are available from employers and FHSAs/Health Boards or directly from the pensions agencies. BMA members can obtain guidance notes from local BMA offices; more complicated queries are dealt with by the BMA superannuation department.

Personal pension plans (PPPs)

As retirement approaches, your PPP provider will be able to tell you the value of your investment fund and the amount of pension and lump sum that is likely to accrue from it. Remember that you do not have to take your PPP at the same time as the NHS pension and that the level of interest rates prevailing as you approach retirement will be a significant factor (the higher the interest rates, the higher the pension, and vice versa).

It is also important to remember that it is not necessary to take your pension from the company that sold you the personal pension (your PPP provider) and that in many cases it would be a mistake to do so. You are perfectly entitled to take the 'open market' option and to use your investment fund to buy a pension from whichever company is offering the most competitive annuity rates at the time of your retirement.

Further details are given in Chapter 6. If in doubt, you may wish to seek independent financial advice.

Investing the NHS pension scheme lump sum, and other investments

This subject has been covered in Chapters 7 and 13.

As retirement approaches, it is advisable to obtain an estimate of what your NHS pension scheme lump sum is likely to be (see above) and to consider this, along with any other investments you may have, in relation to your overall financial position. You may wish to use some of the lump sum to finance a particular purchase you have been planning to make. Once such a decision is made, a balance has to be struck between a need for continuing income in retirement over and above the NHS pension and a need for capital investment, which should generate *future* income or expenditure.

These decisions will need to take account of whether you are retiring before, at or after the State retirement age (see below). If you retire before this age, there may be a need for additional income until the State pension becomes payable. Again, this is an area in which sound, reliable and independent financial advice is important.

State benefits

Whether or not the full State pension is payable depends upon whether you have a full national insurance contribution record. Many people will have a shortfall of contributions because they started paying these late (doctors, for example, do not qualify until at least age 23), because of career breaks or even because they have not lived in the UK throughout their full working life. Different rules apply to those women who have opted to pay the married woman's reduced rate of contribution. Further details are given in Chapter 17.

You can plan ahead and find out what your State pension is going to be by obtaining form BR19 from your local Department of Social Security or Benefits Agency office, completing it and sending it off to the Pensions Forecast Unit in Newcastle Upon Tyne (*see* Appendix A).

How much money will I need when I retire?

There is understandable concern on the part of many people as they approach retirement that their income will drop substantially when they retire and that they will not have enough money to allow them to live as comfortably as they would wish. This concern is often justified. Poverty amongst the elderly continues to be a major problem in the UK, and, no doubt, if the State pension (and/or other State benefits) is the only source of retirement income, hardship is virtually inevitable. However, for those who have spent their career in the NHS, or with some other employer with a good occupational pension scheme, the picture is not so bleak. In fact, people often underestimate the likely standard of living that they can achieve once retired. A combination of an NHS and State pension, together with the prospect of some income from other sources (eg personal pensions, investments or part-time work) can add up to a very satisfactory level of income overall.

People also sometimes overlook the other side of the equation, namely the reduction in expenditure or outgoings that occurs on retirement. Such savings can accrue in many ways after retirement; for example, many of the costs associated with working *per se* will largely disappear or be substantially reduced.

- NHS pension scheme contributions are no longer payable.

- National insurance contributions are no longer payable.

- Because income is lower, the amount and proportion of income tax payable may be lower.

- Commuting costs will disappear.

- Other ancillary costs, such as for work-related clothing, will be reduced.

At the same time as work-related costs disappear, savings will become available in many areas:

- many types of concession will be available, for instance concessionary fares on public transport

- off-peak and/or senior citizen prices will be available for holidays, entertainment, etc.

Retirement, or the years immediately preceding it, may also be a time when the costs of a mortgage or child rearing will finally have been completed (or at least the worst should be over!). The end of these major financial commitments can make a big impact.

For many people, therefore, the financial position in retirement will be quite satisfactory; it may even bring increased prosperity and the opportunities to enjoy these years of leisure and activity, secure in the knowledge that a reasonable standard of living can be maintained.

Making a will

Although many people make a will before they retire, some do not. It is essential to do so to ensure that your assets are left to those people you wish to have them. It is not sufficient to assume that your spouse will receive everything on your death. This may not always be the case, for example if you have children.

A will also presents an opportunity to nominate a person to look after your estate after your death, which can be particularly important if you have children under the age of 18. A will may also help you to avoid inheritance tax or reduce the amount you need to pay (see below).

It is possible to write your own will if your particular circumstances are not complicated. Forms are available from stationers. However, it may be safer to use a solicitor or a specialist will-writing company. The law in Scotland relating to wills is significantly different from the law in England and Wales.

Inheritance tax

You may not wish to make any plans about inheritance tax. Any savings will, after all, not accrue until after your death. You may even feel that it is not unreasonable for such a tax to be payable, or you may feel that your estate is not likely to be large enough to worry about.

However, it is surprisingly easy for an estate to be affected by inheritance tax, and if you want your heirs to benefit as much as possible from your assets, inheritance tax planning is certainly worth considering. Such planning has potential pitfalls as you can lose control of your assets and create financial difficulties for yourself. Perhaps the most important consideration is to ensure that you do not create unnecessary difficulties for your old age.

The first £150 000 of your estate is tax free, ie there is a nil rate tax band. There is also no tax on assets given, or left when you die, to your husband or wife. In addition, certain gifts are exempt from inheritance tax, and certain other types of gift are exempt if made more than seven years before your death. These exempt gifts do not count towards the £150 000 tax-free limit. It may be possible to reduce the scale of inheritance tax by making lifetime gifts, distributing wealth between husband and wife, using your will to make gifts, making arrangements within trusts or making special arrangements for ownership of your home. However, these are complicated matters which need to be considered carefully on the basis of professional advice.

Housing

To move or not to move?

The grass is always greener on the other side, and retirement is a tempting opportunity to move to an idyllic locality, perhaps even to another (warmer and sunnier) climate.

Many people have made such a move successfully and it may well be a sensible option to pursue, particularly if you have been more or less tied to your present locality by your work. A move may also take you closer to family, as well as to an area you prefer.

However, there is also much to be said in favour of staying where you are, at least until you have fully adjusted to the new way of life that retirement brings. This is particularly true if your family is nearby, but other considerations are also important. You may actually like the area and house you live in, feel part of a community, know and enjoy the parks, shops, pubs, cinemas, library, church and other amenities. These things are important to happiness and health and should not be given up lightly.

Altering your house

If you do stay, you may feel that the house is too big or old, or too expensive to heat and maintain. Houses can be adapted and improved, and it is a good idea to think about these aspects before your income drops. Some improvements, such as heating insulation, can actually save money in the long term, as well as adding to your general comfort. Remember also that you will be spending much more time in the house and it may not seem quite as big after retirement as it did when you were working.

Security

Fortunately, crime against older people is not common, despite the unfortunate publicity it often attracts. Most burglaries are opportunist and over very quickly, and some simple precautions can substantially reduce the risk. Doors and windows should have proper locks and a burglar alarm is a useful deterrent. A neighbourhood watch scheme may be operating in your area.

For more detailed and expert advice as you prepare for retirement, ask the crime prevention officer at your local police station to visit you and inspect your home. This is a service the police are very willing to provide.

You may also wish to review your house insurance – buildings and contents – to ensure that it is at the appropriate level and that you are getting the best deal possible.

Income from your house

A considerable number of home owners in retirement can be described as 'housing rich, income poor', and there are ways in which this 'rich housing' can be used to raise income levels.

Perhaps the most obvious is to sell a large house and move to a smaller one. Alternatively, there may be the possibility of staying in the large house but earning rental income from lodgers.

More complicated methods are also available, some of which can be perfectly safe and allow you to raise capital on your home while still living in it.

A mortgage annuity plan enables you to take out a mortgage on your home and use the money raised to purchase an annuity. Part of the annuity income is then used to pay off the interest on the mortgage and the remainder is available as regular income. With this method you retain ownership of the house and you or your heirs benefit from any future increases in its value. The loan is repaid on your death, or earlier if you move, from the sale of the house.

A home reversion scheme involves actually selling your house but retaining the right to live in it for the rest of your life at a nominal rent. This income can be paid as a lump sum or you can purchase an annuity. However, with this type of plan, the value placed on the house is always very considerably below the market value. You lose the benefit of future increases in value, and you cannot of course leave the house to your heirs or sell it if you wish to move later on.

With any type of scheme involving the raising of money on your home, caution is essential and sound, and genuinely independent legal and financial advice is advisable.

Your partner

The majority of people live with a husband, wife or partner. For them, your retirement is also a time of considerable readjustment, and it is important that they play a major part in the preparations for retirement. Your partner may not be used to having you around the house all day and will have developed ways of living and activities that will inevitably be disturbed.

Seeing a lot more of one another can in itself create tension. Everyone has a need for space and for time to themselves. These aspects need to be considered and discussed as a couple, so that you fully appreciate each other's position and can make any necessary arrangements to smooth the transition.

Caring for elderly parents

Many people preparing for their retirement also have responsibilities for the care of their parents. This is increasingly the case as life expectancy continues to improve.

Although in some cases the responsibility is dealt with by having the parents live with you, for most people the preference of parents and children alike is that people live in their own homes for as long as possible. In this case, the home can be made safer and easier to use in a variety of ways.

When living at home is no longer possible or desired, sheltered housing may be a good alternative. This can be purchased or rented. It usually involves purpose-built housing with a warden, alarm system, communal garden and sitting room and optional meals.

Help is available from a number of sources in caring for elderly parents:

- local authorities provide certain services, including meals on wheels and home helps

- your parents' GP may have useful advice. If nursing care is needed, a nurse may be able to visit regularly

- other specialist assistance is available from social workers and health visitors

- Age Concern (see Appendix A) can assist with advice and information

- local voluntary organizations, contacted through the local Citizens Advice Bureau, often provide practical assistance to elderly people.

Benefits are also available from the State. Attendance allowance is paid to people who need almost constant care. This is tax free and is not means tested. Disability living allowance may also be payable. The local Department of Social Security office or Benefits Agency can provide full details of the benefits that are available. Alternatively, you can use the free telephone advice numbers listed in Chapter 17.

Health

Chapter 19 discusses health in retirement in some detail. However, it is not necessary to wait until retirement age to start reassessing your health and taking steps to improve your long-term health prospects. All pre-retirement training courses (see below) include health issues as a most important element. The process of preparing for retirement provides an ideal opportunity for a period of quiet reassessment and reflection. Many people, particularly those working in the highly demanding and stressful environment of the modern NHS, become so wrapped up in the task of looking after the health needs of others that they neglect their own. This is true even of doctors. Recent studies have shown that, across a range of health indicators, GPs are not as healthy as their peers in other professions. When preparing for retirement, there is an ideal opportunity to put this right.

Pre-retirement courses

The Pre-Retirement Association of Great Britain and Northern Ireland (see Appendix A) celebrated its thirtieth anniversary in 1994. It is an independent national organization specializing in retirement planning and can provide details of courses that are available. You should also check with your employers in case they are running courses for their staff or are willing to finance your attendance at a course. The best courses will usually encourage you to bring your spouse or partner; retirement planning is very much a joint exercise.

In choosing a course, caution is called for in respect of the financial planning section. Investment decisions should not be made without taking financial advice that is genuinely independent.

Doctors who are BMA members are able to attend pre-retirement courses run by the BMA superannuation department in conjunction with the Pre-Retirement Association. The courses are available to doctors aged 57 or over (55 or over if space permits) and are run on a rotating basis in each NHS region, as well as in Wales, Scotland and Northern Ireland. Courses cover the following subjects:

- attitudes to retirement
- the NHS pension scheme
- financial planning

- health in retirement
- state benefits
- leisure.

The present cost of the BMA courses in 1995 is £60 for a doctor and £90 for a couple. Spouses are encouraged to attend.

The financial planning talk is given by BMA Services Ltd (see Appendix A), which has been established in order to provide independent financial advice to doctors who are BMA members.

Appendix A   Organizations active in the world of pensions and retirement

The NHS pension scheme: pensions agencies

England and Wales
  NHS Pensions Agency
  Hesketh House
  200–220 Broadway
  Fleetwood
  Lancashire
  FY7 8LG
  Tel: (0253) 774774

Scotland
  Scottish Office Pensions Agency
  St Margaret's House
  151 London Road
  Edinburgh
  EH8 7TG
  Tel: 031-244 3585 or 031-556 8400

Northern Ireland
  Health and Personal Social Services
  Superannuation Branch (HRD 6)
  Waterside House
  75 Duke Street
  Waterside
  Londonderry
  BT47 1FP
  Tel: (0504) 319000

General practitioners: Northern Ireland

Central Services Agency
25 Adelaide Street
Belfast
BT2 8FD
Tel: (0232) 324431
Note: Administers GPs' pay and liaises with Superannuation Branch in Londonderry (details above)

General dental practitioners

Dental Practice Board
Compton Place Road
Eastbourne
East Sussex
BN20 8AD
Tel: (0323) 417000

NHS pension scheme: payment of benefits

The Paymaster
(Paymaster General's Office)
Sutherland House
Russell Way
Crawley
West Sussex
RH10 1UH
Tel: (0293) 560999

Additional voluntary contributions (AVCs)

The Equitable Life Assurance Society
PO Box 183
Walton Street
Aylesbury
Buckinghamshire
HP21 7QW
Tel: (0296) 384040

Other pension schemes

Universities
    Universities Superannuation Scheme
    Richmond House
    Rumford Place
    Liverpool
    L3 9FD
    Tel: 051-236 3173

Civil Service
    Principal Civil Service pension scheme
    Civil Service Pension Division of the Treasury
    Alencon Link
    Basingstoke
    Hampshire
    RG21 1JB
    Tel: (0256) 29222

Armed forces pension scheme

    Royal Navy:
    Director of Naval Pay and Pensions
    Ministry of Defence
    HMS Centurion
    Grange Road
    Gosport
    Hampshire
    PO13 9XA
    Tel: (0705) 822351

    Army:
    Army Pensions Office
    Kentigern House
    65 Brown Street
    Glasgow
    G2 8EX
    Tel: 041-224 2681

    Royal Air Force:
    RAF Pensions
    RAF Insworth

Gloucester
GL3 1EZ
Tel: (0452) 712612

Medical Research Council

Medical Research Council Pension Scheme
20 Park Crescent
London
W1N 4AL
Tel: 071-636 5422

Ombudsman

Pensions Ombudsman
11 Belgrave Road
London
SW1V 1RB
Tel: 071-834 9144

Advisory service (complaints)

Occupational Pensions Advisory Service
OPAS
11 Belgrave Road
London
SW1V 1RB
Tel: 071-233 8080

State pension forecast

Benefits Agency
RPFA Unit
Newcastle Pensions Directorate
Newcastle Upon Tyne
NE98 1YX

Professional associations and trade unions

British Medical Association
Superannuation Department
BMA House
Tavistock Square
London
WC1H 9JP
Tel: 071-383 6166

Royal College of Nursing
20 Cavendish Square
London
W1M 0AB
Tel: 071-409 3333

British Dental Association
64 Wimpole Street
London
W1M 8AL
Tel: 071-935 0875

UNISON
1 Mabledon Place
London
WC1H 9AJ
Tel: 071-388 2366

Chartered Society of Physiotherapy
14 Bedford Row
London
WC1R 4ED
Tel: 071-242 1941

Royal College of Midwives
15 Mansfield Street
London
W1M 0BE
Tel: 071-580 6523

British Orthoptic Society
Tavistock House North
Tavistock Square
London
WC1H 9HX
Tel: 071-387 7992

Regulatory authorities

Personal Investment Authority
Pensions Unit
1 London Wall 5th Floor
London
EC2Y 5EA
Tel: 071-417 7001

Securities and Investment Board
Gavrelle House
2–14 Bunhill Row
London
EC1Y 8RA
Tel: 071-638 1240

Financial Intermediaries, Managers and Brokers Regulatory Association
(FIMBRA)
Hertsmere House
Hertsmere Road
London
E14 4AB
Tel: 071-895 8579

Life Assurance and Unit Trust Regulatory Organisation (LAUTRO)
Centre Point
103 New Oxford Street
London
WC1A 1QH
Tel: 071-379 0444

Investment Management Regulatory Organisation (IMRO)
Broadwalk House
6 Appold Street
London
EC2A 2AA
Tel: 071-628 6022

Government bodies

Occupational Pensions Board (OPB)
PO Box 2EE
Newcastle Upon Tyne
NE99 2EE
Tel: 091-225 6414

Pensions Registry
(traces past pension entitlements)
PO Box 1NN
Newcastle Upon Tyne
NE99 1NN
Tel: 091-225 6393/4

Pension Schemes Office
(Inland Revenue)
Lynwood Road
Thames Ditton
Surrey
KT7 0DP
Tel: 081-398 4242

Benefits Agency
(Department of Social Security)
Publicity Register (leaflets, etc)
4th Floor
1 Trevelyan Square
Boar Lane
Leeds
LS1 6EB
Tel: (0645) 540000

Financial advice

BMA Services Ltd
BMA House
Tavistock Square
London
WC1H 9JP
Tel: 071-387 4311

RCN Membership Services
Regent House
Hubert Road
Brentwood
Essex
CM14 4QQ
Tel: (01277) 261630

Asset Financial Planning (Age Concern)
Freepost
PO Box 106
37 Broad Street
Bristol
BS99 7YJ
Tel: (0272) 263822

Preparation for retirement

Pre-retirement Association
NODUS Centre
University Campus
Guildford
Surrey
GU2 5RX
Tel: (0483) 39323

Leisure, voluntary work, education and general information
National Association of Pension Funds (NAPF)

12–18 Grosvenor Gardens
London
SW1W 0DH
Tel: 071-730 0585

Age Concern

England
   Astral House
   1268 London Road
   London
   SW16 4ER
   Tel: 081-79 8000

Wales
   4th Floor
   1 Cathedral Road
   Cardiff
   CF1 9SD
   Tel: (0222) 371566

Scotland
   54a Fountainbridge
   Edinburgh
   EH3 9PT
   Tel: 031-228 5656

Northern Ireland
   3 Lower Crescent
   Belfast
   BT7 1NR
   Tel: (0232) 245729

Voluntary work

REACH
89 Southwark Street
London
SE1 0HD
Tel: 071-928 0452

Citizens Advice Bureaux
115–123 Pentonville Road
London
N1 9LZ
Tel: 071-833 2181

National Council for Voluntary Organisations
26 Bedford Square
London
WC1B 3HU
Tel: 071-636 4066

Directory of British Associations
(Consult this in your local library)

Education

Open University
Central Enquiry Service
PO Box 200
Walton Hall
Milton Keynes
MK7 6YZ
Tel: (0908) 653231

University of the Third Age
U3A National Office
1 Stockwell Green
London
SW9 9JF
Tel: 071-737 2541

National Institute of Adult Continuing Education
19b De Montfort Street
Leicester
LE1 7GE
Tel: (0533) 551451

Travel

SAGA Holidays
Freepost

Folkestone
Kent
CT20 1BR
Tel: (0800) 300 500

World Association for Disability and Rehabilitation (RADAR)
Unit 12
City Forum
250 City Road
London
EC1V 8AF
Tel: 071-250 3222

The Automobile Association publishes *Traveller's Guide for the Disabled* and the *World Wheelchair Traveller*

Appendix B Early retirement factors

Age	Complete months											
	0	1	2	3	4	5	6	7	8	9	10	11
Pensions												
50	0.599	0.601	0.604	0.606	0.608	0.610	0.612	0.614	0.616	0.618	0.620	0.622
51	0.624	0.627	0.629	0.631	0.634	0.636	0.638	0.640	0.643	0.645	0.647	0.650
52	0.652	0.654	0.657	0.660	0.662	0.665	0.667	0.670	0.672	0.675	0.677	0.680
53	0.682	0.685	0.688	0.691	0.694	0.696	0.699	0.702	0.705	0.708	0.711	0.713
54	0.716	0.719	0.723	0.726	0.729	0.732	0.735	0.738	0.742	0.745	0.748	0.751
55	0.754	0.758	0.761	0.765	0.768	0.772	0.775	0.779	0.782	0.785	0.789	0.792
56	0.796	0.800	0.803	0.807	0.811	0.815	0.818	0.822	0.826	0.830	0.833	0.837
57	0.841	0.845	0.849	0.853	0.857	0.861	0.865	0.869	0.873	0.878	0.882	0.886
58	0.890	0.894	0.899	0.903	0.907	0.912	0.916	0.921	0.925	0.929	0.934	0.938
59	0.943	0.947	0.952	0.957	0.962	0.966	0.971	0.976	0.981	0.986	0.990	0.995
Lump sums												
50	0.747	0.749	0.751	0.753	0.755	0.756	0.758	0.760	0.762	0.764	0.766	0.767
51	0.769	0.771	0.773	0.775	0.777	0.779	0.780	0.782	0.784	0.786	0.788	0.790
52	0.792	0.794	0.796	0.798	0.800	0.801	0.803	0.805	0.807	0.809	0.811	0.813
53	0.815	0.817	0.819	0.821	0.823	0.825	0.827	0.829	0.831	0.833	0.835	0.837
54	0.839	0.841	0.843	0.845	0.847	0.849	0.851	0.854	0.856	0.858	0.860	0.862
55	0.864	0.866	0.868	0.870	0.872	0.874	0.877	0.879	0.881	0.883	0.885	0.887
56	0.889	0.892	0.894	0.896	0.898	0.900	0.902	0.905	0.907	0.909	0.911	0.913
57	0.916	0.918	0.920	0.922	0.925	0.927	0.929	0.932	0.934	0.936	0.938	0.941
58	0.943	0.945	0.948	0.950	0.952	0.955	0.957	0.959	0.962	0.964	0.966	0.969
59	0.971	0.973	0.976	0.978	0.981	0.983	0.985	0.988	0.990	0.993	0.995	0.998

Example: someone retiring at the age of 57 years and 9 months would receive 87.8% of the pension that had built up at that age and 93.6% of the lump sum built up by that age.

Index